Urodynamic Testing After Spinal Cord Injury

Jean Jacques Wyndaele
Apichana Kovindha

Urodynamic Testing After Spinal Cord Injury

A Practical Guide

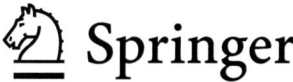 Springer

Jean Jacques Wyndaele
University of Antwerp
Antwerp
Belgium

Apichana Kovindha
Rehabilitation Medicine
Chiang Mai University
Chiang Mai
Thailand

ISBN 978-3-319-54899-9   ISBN 978-3-319-54900-2   (eBook)
DOI 10.1007/978-3-319-54900-2

Library of Congress Control Number: 2017944915

Printed on acid-free paper

This Springer imprint is published by Springer Nature
The registered company is Springer International Publishing AG
The registered company address is: Gewerbestrasse 11, 6330 Cham, Switzerland

Preface

In this handbook, we aim to give a practical guide for urodynamic investigation/testing (UDT) in individuals who have suffered from a spinal cord injury (SCI). It is universally acknowledged that this type of investigation can be valuable and most international guidelines consider it mandatory in patients with neurogenic bladder dysfunction. Performing UDT in a clinical setting seems complicated for those unfamiliar with it. However, concerns can be overcome with proper knowledge of indications, of techniques, and of correct interpretation. This is the scope of this book: to offer all involved evidence-based knowledge of applicability and clinical value but also of limitations. It will permit to acquire the skills needed for a proper application and an accurate interpretation of the results, helping to make an informed decision on treatment options. This will, without doubt, benefit the SCI individuals under care. We neither aim to write a book including all data from research nor plan to deliver a complete overview of UDT in general. Most of what is presented here is based on strong expert opinions from a vast experience gathered during decades of urodynamic testing in SCI individuals in different parts of the world. A high number of UDT tracings from clinical practice permit to gain valuable and specific knowledge.

Antwerp, Belgium   Jean Jacques Wyndaele, M.D.
Chiang Mai, Thailand   Apichana Kovindha, M.D.

Contents

Abbreviations

AD	Autonomic dysreflexia
ASIA	American Spinal Injury Association
BP	Blood pressure
CIC	Clean intermittent catheterization
CISC	Clean intermittent self-catheterization
DSD	Detrusor sphincter dyssynergia
DSS	Detrusor sphincter synergia
EI	End infusion
EMG	Electromyography
FD/FDV	First desire to void
FSF	First sensation of filling
ISCOS	International Spinal Cord Society
ICS	International Continence Society
LEMS	Lower extremity motor score
LUT	Lower urinary tract
ND	Normal desire to void
NDO	Neurogenic detrusor overactivity
Pabd	Abdominal pressure
Pdet	Detrusor pressure
Pura	Urethral pressure
Pves	Vesical pressure
PVR	Post-void residual
Q/Qura	Urine flow rate
SCI	Spinal cord injury/lesion
SD/SDV	Strong desire to void
SI	Start infusion
UDT	Urodynamic investigation/testing
UEMS	Upper extremity motor score
USG	Ultrasonography
UTI	Urinary tract infection
VCUG	Voiding cystourethrogram
VUR	Vesicoureteral reflux

Introduction

Evaluating the function of the lower urinary tract (LUT), disturbed by a neurological pathology, consists of compiling clinical data and technical investigations in order to get an as complete as possible idea of what happens in the LUT during filling and during voiding. When done in individuals who suffered from a traumatic or non-traumatic SCI, urodynamic findings should be included in the overall neurologic evaluation.

Several data sets have been developed to make such task easier. Performing investigations based on the data proposed in the data sets will make them more easy to understand, more easy to standardise while permitting a good communication between different health care professionals.

Neurological deficits after SCI have been traditionally classified using the AIS (American Spinal Injury Association /ISCOS Impairment Scale) [1]. The scale identifies level and completeness of the lesion based on detailed clinical testing of the somatomotor and somatosensory systems. The AIS also indicates, to a certain level, the changes that may have occurred in the autonomic functions, but a more specific and selective evaluation is needed.

The urodynamic functions of the LUT after SCI are different in every individual. The LUT dysfunction is potentially dangerous and can lead to severe symptoms and complications. To prevent such complications, urodynamic testing, so far the best available diagnosis, is mandatory as it is the only objective measure showing how bladder, bladder neck and urethral sphincter probably work and how the interaction is between the three structures.

When the UDT is done with proper indication, best technique and objective/critical interpretation of the measurements, a clear picture will become available of what is and what is not present in the activity of the LUT in this particular individual.

Technical urodynamics also have limitations and these should be acknowledged and looked for.

J.J. Wyndaele, A. Kovindha, *Urodynamic Testing After Spinal Cord Injury*, DOI 10.1007/978-3-319-54900-2_1

Physiology and Pathophysiology

2

An overview of the physiology of the LUT function is indispensable to understand how changes occur after SCI. It will help us interpret data from urodynamic tests correctly. The innervations and functions of the LUT are given in Table 2.1 and Fig. 2.1. One should acquire this basic knowledge to be able to understand what follows.

Table 2.1 Overview of functions of the sympathetic, the parasympathetic and the somatic nerves in the LUT, and the spinal cord level which they relate to

	Sympathetic Spinal cord T10–L2	Parasympathetic Spinal cord S2–S4	Somatic Spinal cord S3–S5
Neurotransmitters	Noradrenaline	Acetylcholine	
Bladder (β3 receptors)	−		
Bladder (M3 receptors)		+	
Bladder neck (α1)	+		
External US	Exp	Exp	+
Sensation in LUT	+	+	+

US urethral sphincter, *Exp* mostly from animal experiments. − = inhibition; + = stimulation

© Springer International Publishing AG 2017
J.J. Wyndaele, A. Kovindha, *Urodynamic Testing After Spinal Cord Injury*,
DOI 10.1007/978-3-319-54900-2_2

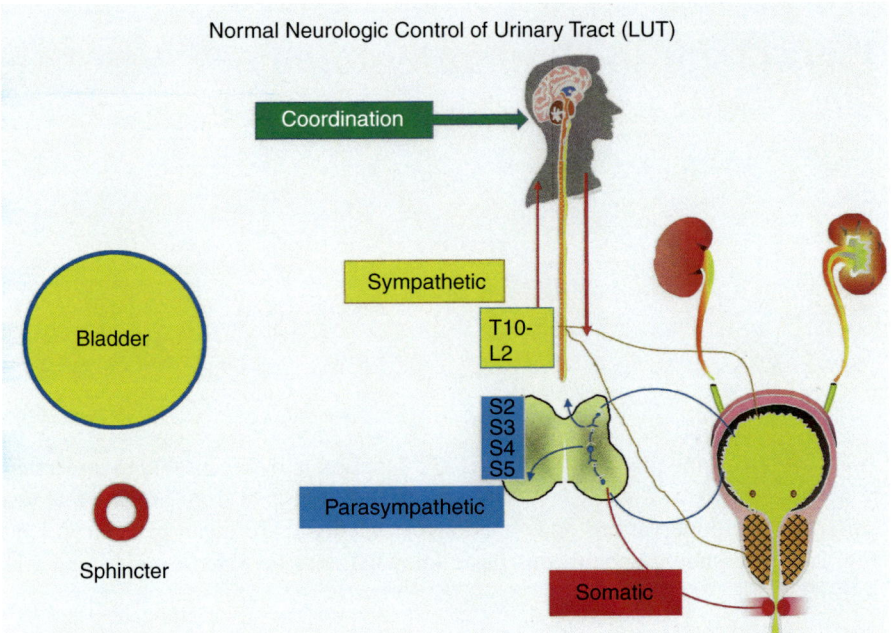

Fig. 2.1 Innervation of the LUT and central control mechanisms. From T10 to L2 the sympathetic control runs through the hypogastric nerves. From S2 to S5 the innervation runs through the pelvic (parasympathetic control) and the pudendal nerves (somatic innervation of the external sphincter and pelvic floor muscles). Sensory information runs through all peripheral nerves and the spinal cord

2.1   Normal Bladder Function

In normal conditions the bladder has an average maximum capacity of 500 ml, with a large variability between individuals. The filling through diuresis happens at a constant rate of 1–10 ml/min from right and left kidney. The bladder wall has the ability to adapt to an increasing filling volume, if such filling is done at a physiological rate. Muscular, neurological and local extensibility mechanisms play a role in keeping the pressure low while the bladder is filled: the bladder is "compliant". Consequence is that the pressure inside the bladder hardly rises, in normal conditions, between empty and full.

During bladder filling, neural information is sent up to the brain and at some level of filling a sensation develops. During urodynamic filling the first sensation of filling (FSF) may occur at about 40% of bladder capacity. This sensation remains unnoticed in daily life but can be reported during UDT when the attention is focused on LUT events. Further filling elicits the first desire to void at around 60–70% of bladder capacity and a strong desire to void at maximum capacity [2].

In healthy persons, no bladder muscle (also called detrusor muscle) contraction with intravesical pressure rise is found during the filling phase and the bladder neck remains closed while the external urethral sphincter contraction increases gradually to maintain urethral closure mechanism and prevent incontinence/leakage.

When a strong desire to void (SDV) makes voiding necessary, the micturition mechanism is started from the brain—a sensation of start of voiding is felt, the contraction of the sphincter ends, the bladder muscle builds up a continuous contraction and urine outflow is seen. Through the central co-ordination, the sphincter remains open during the entire bladder contraction = detrusor-sphincter synergy (DSS). The opening of the bladder neck during voiding results probably from less sympathetic stimuli and from the pulling upwards of the bladder neck funnel by the bladder muscle fibres extending down in the urethra.

2.2 Acute Period After SCI

When an acute SCI occurs, the first period, known as spinal shock, starts and its duration varies from days to months. During spinal shock, spinal reflexes are inactive with a non-contractile bladder as a consequence. Bladder drainage with an indwelling catheter or intermittent catheterization (after stabilization of the cardiovascular unbalance and the restoration of a rhythmic diuresis pattern) helps to avoid overdistension and to keep the elasticity and consequently contractibility of the bladder wall unharmed. In this stage, the UDT shows no bladder activity, no pressure rise during filling phase, and no desire to void. The bladder neck most frequently remains closed. The striated urethral sphincter will keep an intrinsic activity, normal urethral pressure until it restarts its reflex function again [3].

When the spinal shock resolves, the consequences of SCI on the LUT function become more clear. These depend on the level and the extent of the lesion.

2.3 Suprasacral Lesion

A lesion above the sacral cord (Fig. 2.2) corresponds with spine lesion above thoracic 10. The spinal reflex pathways of the bladder, bladder neck and urethral sphincter remain active. Coordination between bladder and sphincter is lost. The bladder muscle (detrusor) can start involuntary contraction related to the grade of bladder filling or another stimulus such as tapping or touching the suprapubic area. Desire to void is absent though other symptoms may indicate bladder contraction and/or grade of bladder filling, e.g. undefined general signs, autonomic reactions such as sweating, piloerection (goose bump skin above the level of lesion). If a lesion is incomplete, the desire to void may be preserved.

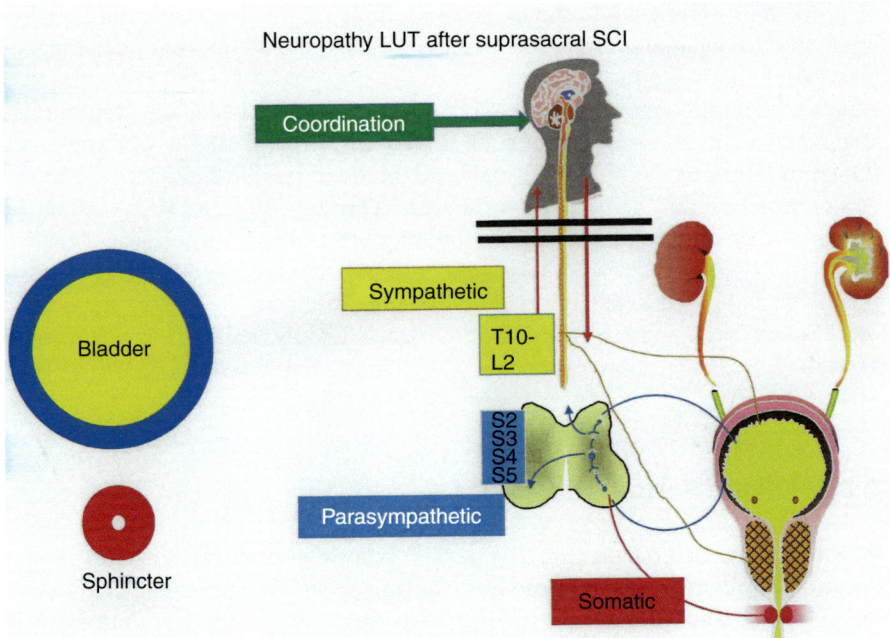

Fig. 2.2 Lesion at the thoracic spinal cord *above* the innervation of the LUT, gives loss of cerebral control and coordination, causing neurogenic overactivity of both bladder and external urethral sphincter *(depicted as bold wall of bladder and sphincter at the left side)*

Many patients have flaccid lower extremities while the bladder and the sphincter are spastic or overactive.

2.4 Sacral-Subsacral Lesion

Lesion at the sacral cord (Fig. 2.3) can destruct the bladder motor pathways. The sphincter may be neurologically preserved or may become denervated and thus the loss of detrusor and/or sphincter contractility depends on the extent of the neurologic destruction. With the sacral cord (conus medullaris) positioned at spine level L1–L2, lesions at the lower thoracic to higher lumbar vertebrae may result in preservation of part of the innervation or loss of such innervation. It is very difficult in these cases to predict from clinical data what the LUT functions will be.

The bladder neck function depends on the intact activity of the sympathetic nerves (hypogastric nerves). A lesion can occur with spinal fracture at the level of the sympathetic outflow. When completely destroyed, a continuous open bladder neck may be seen.

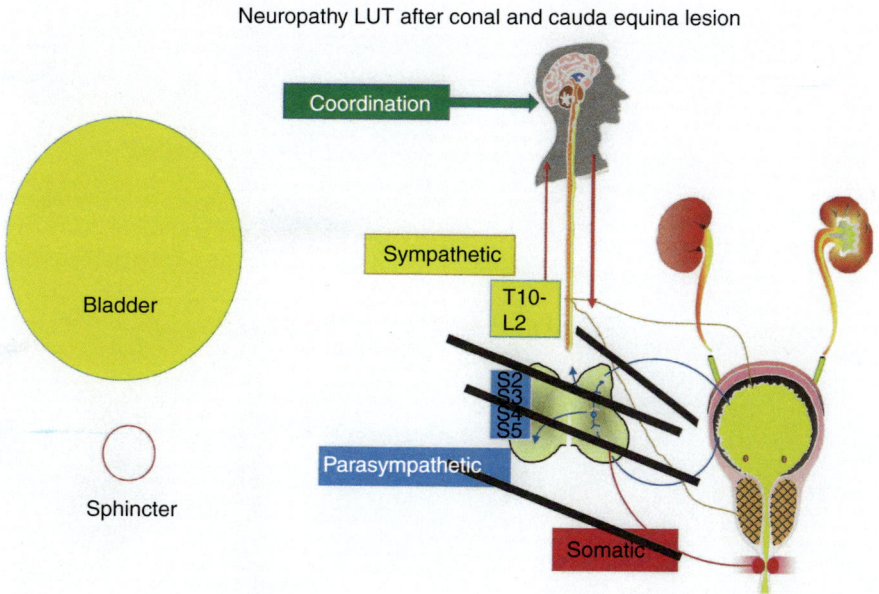

Fig. 2.3 Lesions at the sacral cord and cauda equina, causing acontractility of both bladder and external urethral sphincter *(depicted as thin bladder and sphincter at the left side).*

Diagnosis of Neurogenic LUT Dysfunction after SCI

3

Information on the remaining innervation of the LUT after SCI should be acquired from history taking and clinical neurological examination. How many investigations are needed depends on each individual patient, the stage of SCI management (acute phase, post-acute rehabilitation phase, long-term phase of follow-up) (Table 3.1). This will also help determine which tests should be done and when, and if a test should be repeated.

Table 3.1 Urological investigations to be done during the acute, the spinal post-acute rehab, and follow-up/long-term phases

	Acute phase	Post-acute rehab phase	Post discharge Follow-up/long-term phase
General history	+	+	+
More specific/relevant history		+	+
Physical examination	+	+	+
Neurological examination	+	+	When indicated
Urine tests	+	+	+
Blood analysis	+	When indicated	
Urodynamic testing (UDT)		+	When indicated
Imaging	+	+	+
Specialized urological tests	When indicated		

+, recommended to do

© Springer International Publishing AG 2017   9
J.J. Wyndaele, A. Kovindha, *Urodynamic Testing After Spinal Cord Injury*,
DOI 10.1007/978-3-319-54900-2_3

3.1   Patient History

Primary general history taking should be started with a quick overview of the patient's condition: age, gender, race, general condition, possibility to communicate with reference to language, cognitive abilities, functional level, motivation, cooperation and psychological status.

Further history taking should explore previous diseases of the urinary tract, drug intake, techniques of bladder drainage used and eventual problems which occurred, urinary tract infection (UTI) and other LUT complications. An assessment of sexual, and bowel functions should also be included as there is an important overlap of innervation of the different pelvic organs, and a strong interaction between them [4].

In a chronic stage, signs and symptoms related to storage and voiding, and possible complications such as fever, haematuria, pain, inflammation in the pelvic region, autonomic dysreflexia (AD) and more, have to be asked.

3.2   Urinary Diary (Frequency/Volume Chart)

In the acute stage, diuresis will be followed daily by the indwelling catheter drainage. A frequency/volume chart is useful in the rehabilitation phase and during follow-up, in different types of bladder emptying. Desire to void, time and volume for each voiding or catheterization, 24 h diuresis volume, fluid intake, leakage with subjective estimate of quantity or by weighing of diapers, should be assessed and recorded. If catheterization is done, post void residual urine (PVR) should be measured.

Filling in a frequency/volume chart during 3 consecutive days is a good compromise between getting proper data and keeping the patient/carer compliant. In a patient who performs only intermittent catheterization, the information of a frequency/volume chart may be valuable to know fluctuations in diuresis, to determine which catheterization frequency should be adopted and if a full bladder elicits sensation.

3.3   Questionnaires

The international spinal cord injury data sets such as the International LUT Function Basic Spinal Cord Injury data set, the International Urinary Tract Imaging Basic Spinal cord Injury data set and the International Urodynamic Spinal Cord Injury basic data set are clinically very helpful and are a necessity for research *(see Chap. 18 Data Sets)*.

To define quality of life, "Qualiveen" has shown a clear merit [5]. A questionnaire evaluating bladder and bowel symptoms together, needs to be evaluated in SCI [6].

3.4   Physical Examination

Physical examination should be done in every SCI patient from the first evaluation, and be repeated over time during rehabilitation and follow-up. Testing bilateral sensation of the perineum for light touch and pinprick, tone/resistance of the anal sphincter against insertion of a finger, voluntary contraction of the anal sphincter/pelvic muscles, reflexes related to parts of the LUT innervations (e.g. cremaster reflex in male, anal reflex, bulbocavernosus reflex), give information on all peripheral nerves and central neurologic structures related to LUT function (Fig. 3.1). The anatomical localization and extent of the neurologic lesion(s) can thus be clinically confirmed.

One should be aware of the limitations of the physical and neurological examination but experience will permit to make them more reliable. Extrapolating the results of the tests to the dysfunction of bladder, bladder neck and urethral sphincter, must be done with caution. Especially in vertebral fracture at T12- L1, it has been proven impossible to predict types of LUT dysfunction. For every level of SCI, the resulting LUT dysfunction can differ between individual patients. Prolapse, inguinal hernia, genital infections, penile and scrotal pathology, meatus pathology and prostate disorders may influence the LUT function and should be looked for.

The neurologic lesion has to be defined according to the International Standards for Neurological Classification of SCI (ISNCSCI), including the neurological level of the lesion and the American Spinal Injury Association Impairment Scale (AIS) [1].

3.5   Laboratory Tests

Urine analysis is an important test from admission, during rehabilitation, when problems occur and in the long term follow up. The interpretation of a urine sample must take into account the technique of bladder emptying, presence of an indwelling catheter, symptoms, previous history and treatment, and confounding diseases.

Blood tests may evaluate general condition, renal function, and may be indicated when inflammation or infection is suspected.

3.6   Tests to Evaluate LUT Functions

Post-void residual urine (PVR) assessed with catheterization provides an accurate volume measurement. It is cheap but invasive. In individuals performing CISC, it is easy to get urine and measure PVR. Ultrasonography (USG) is an alternative technique but needs expensive equipment; Bladder Scan is a specific tool which is also not invasive but not cheap.

What can be considered a "normal" PVR is still a matter of dispute. Amounts above 100 cc are often considered - on expert opinion - enough reason to change the

a   **Sensory dermatomes**

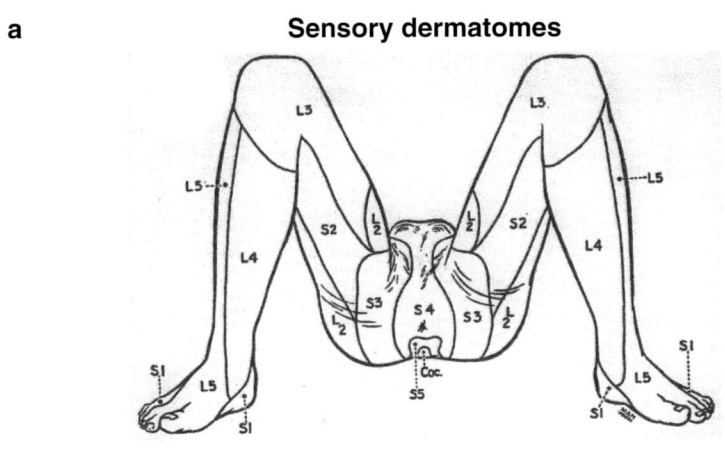

b   **Lumbosacral reflexes**

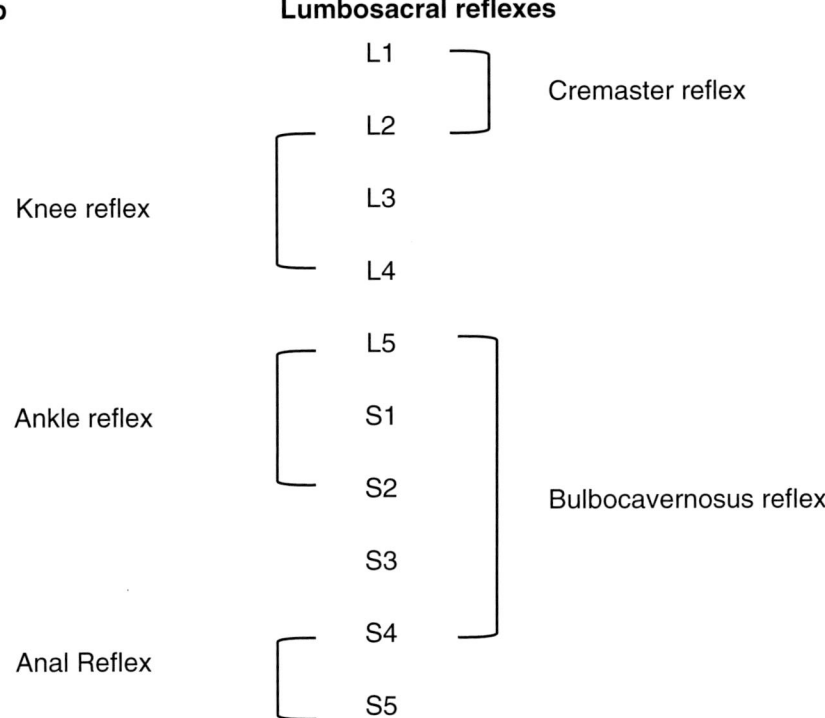

Fig. 3.1 Components of neurological physical examination related to the LUT function after SCI. (**a**) Represents sensory dermatomes, and (**b**) lumbosacral reflexes

bladder emptying technique. The importance of PVR depends on bladder emptying technique, incidence of complications and leakage/urinary incontinence.

Urodynamic investigation (UDT) is an objective measurement of the LUT function, during bladder filling, and voiding or leaking. *It provides more specific data for diagnosis of the neurogenic LUT dysfunction and is recommended for SCI patients who have failure to void and/or failure to store the urine.*

Some SCI individuals report "normal" urination, while UDT shows neurogenic detrusor overactivity (NDO) or voiding with Valsalva.

Techniques of UDT

4

UDT consists of following measurements:

Cystometry is a measurement of pressure in the bladder during bladder filling and is done by introducing a tube into the bladder which is connected to an external pressure measuring device. While the bladder is filled it demonstrates NDO, measures the extensibility of the bladder wall, the pressure point at leakage and can be used to help evaluate filling sensation. When limited resources do not allow purchasing an electronic equipment, a cheap one channel cystometry device permits to gain valuable information. But interpretation is easier when bladder pressure measurement is combined with measurement of intrarectal/intraabdominal pressure as discussed below.

Uroflowmetry measures the flow rate during voiding. It needs voluntary control of voiding which may not be the case in SCI individuals.

Pressure-flow study measures detrusor pressure during voiding. It can assess several functional LUT parameters in patients with other neuropathy but is less easy to perform in many SCI patients who cannot void on command.

Imaging-urodynamic or *video-urodynamic study* under X-rays or with ultrasonography has the great advantage to provide combined functional and anatomical data. Important findings are summarised in the International SCI Basic Urodynamic data set.

Ambulatory UDT is a newer way to follow LUT function during daily activities in the wheelchair, but needs more specialised equipment.

Urethral pressure profile measures urethral pressure over the length of the urethra. It is rarely used in SCI individuals.

> *It is strongly advised to adapt the UDT technique to the neurologic condition after SCI.*

© Springer International Publishing AG 2017

J.J. Wyndaele, A. Kovindha, *Urodynamic Testing After Spinal Cord Injury*,
DOI 10.1007/978-3-319-54900-2_4

Performing UDT

5

5.1   Positioning of the Patient

Choice between supine and sitting position depends on availability of a special table for UDT, and the mobility of the patient. Bedside UDT is possible but less practical when a multichannel electronic device is used.

Pressure development changes with a different position. In any case, a patient should be comfortable, well protected against pressure ulcer development, with material to collect out flow of urine and faeces. The mean duration of a UDT is, transfers included, around 30–45 min, depending on the filling rate.

Neurologic examination and specific manipulation in the lumbosacral area may be needed in some cases, which needs easy access to the genital area and perineum.

5.2   Placing the Measurement Catheters

A bladder pressure catheter must be introduced gently through the urethra so that its openings are well inside the bladder. Preferably a non-anaesthetic lubricant is used to preserve the evaluation of local sensation. Mostly used are small calibre catheters, either special UDT catheters (4–8 Fr) or an ordinary non-hydrophilic catheter Fr 8–10. The choice of material of the catheter will depend on availability, budget, allergy for latex. If spasticity at the sphincter blocks the further insertion of the catheter, extra gel, anaesthetic gel, or rarely stretching of the spastic anal sphincter can help. Difficulty to introduce due to kinking in the bulbar urethra in men, can be overcome with digital support/stretching of the urethra through the rectum, vagina or perineal surface. When no imaging is available, the position of the catheter can be indicated by the outflow of urine, and guided by the length of catheter introduced. In women 7–10 cm and in men 20 cm or more must have passed the external meatus. The catheter connected to the pressure gauge, is securely fixed at the meatus, the perineal area or the thigh. The entire pressure measuring tube should,

© Springer International Publishing AG 2017   17
J.J. Wyndaele, A. Kovindha, *Urodynamic Testing After Spinal Cord Injury*,
DOI 10.1007/978-3-319-54900-2_5

before introduction of the catheter, be filled with filling solution. The pressure measured is "Pves".

A *bowel pressure catheter* is used to measure the rectal/abdominal pressure "Pabd". A catheter with a balloon at the top is inserted through the anal sphincter with lubricant and eventually on a penetrating finger if the anal sphincter is spastic. If a special UDT catheter is not available, a urinary catheter can be used with open end or broad side holes in the proximal part. A balloon is made with a finger cut from a glove or a condom and fixed, covering the proximal holes, around the catheter with a string. When introduced in the rectum its top is protected by a condom. The catheter should be introduced 5–8 cm (if possible) through the anus. If the rectum is filled with stool, the bowel should preferably be emptied. The rectal catheter and its balloon are filled with water and connected to the pressure gauge.

> *If one chooses to prepare the patient for UDT with an enema, it should be applied early enough beforehand (day before) to avoid defecation on the urodynamic table during the test.*

A *urethral pressure catheter* with side holes is used to measure the pressure at the urethral sphincter "Pura". This tube may, together with a filling tube and a bladder pressure measuring tube, be part of a 3 channel catheter.

The catheter is introduced till the side holes are in the bladder, filled with saline and then slowly retracted until the urethral pressure tracing shows a clear pressure rise. This indicates that the holes are at the level of the urethral sphincter. The catheter is fixed to the skin in this position.

5.3   Calibration and Controlling of the Pressure Lines

Zeroing of the transducers can be done with the catheters outside the body, positioned at the level of the bladder, or after introduction and fixation. If done before introduction, Pves and Pabd will show pressures above zero. If done after positioning in the body both traces should start at zero. In both cases Pdet should always start at zero.

Before starting filling with all catheters positioned and connected to the pressure gauges, the patient is asked to cough or in case where this is not feasible, the investigator can push on the lower abdomen. A clear pressure rise related to these actions must be seen in both Pves and Pabd tracings.

If an electronic urodynamic equipment is used with automatic subtraction of Pabd from Pves, providing Pdet, the actions described above must result in no pressure change on the Pdet tracing as the pressure induced in Pves and Pabd should change identically.

5.4 Filling Solution

Sterile saline is used, or a sterile contrast solution if a video-urodynamic test is performed. A bottle or sack with clear marks of volume is preferable, unless one has a system where the volume of fluid used to fill is electronically given through an automatic weighing or other technique. The filling solution can be heated to body temperature or used on room temperature. The results of the UDT may differ somewhat depending on which is used.

5.5 Filling Rate

Continuous filling is mostly used, either by a continuous inflow pump or a valve on the filling tube. Filling rate should be low. But a time factor can also play as in the availability of the UDT room. A good compromise can be filling at 20–50 ml/min in a case where no detrusor overactivity is expected and takes 15–20 min measurement time. Ten to 20 ml/min is preferable when NDO is expected. It will not need more investigation time as the main data of the test will mostly appear at lower bladder capacity.

5.6 Maximum Filling Volume

The filling is stopped at 400–500 ml when no or little pressure develops, in order to avoid over-distension. When NDO occurs, one can decide to stop the filling at the first contraction, if the purpose of the test was mainly to detect NDO.

If more information is needed, the filling can be continued until leakage is noticed or if the pressure becomes regularly higher than 40 cm H_2O.

Different types of pressure development can be seen (*see Chap.* 16).

This approach does not work in cases with massive vesico-renal reflux (VUR), where a large quantity of filling fluid can run to the kidneys keeping the bladder pressure artificially low.

5.7 Electromyography

Electromyography (EMG) of the pelvic floor muscles can give information on striated sphincter behaviour during bladder filling and voiding, and can help make a distinction between different types of DSD. But the EMG activity can be influenced by external and internal factors such as spasticity of the lower limbs, movement of the needle, coughing so that interpretation should be done with some caution. The most direct EMG signal can be obtained by putting a coaxial needle directly in the urethral sphincter, but such positioning is not easy. Alternatives are a needle in another perineal muscle, or surface electrodes put on the perineal skin.

5.8   Imaging

If radiology or ultrasonography (USG) equipment is available during UDT, imaging becomes possible during filling and voiding. A lot of information can be gained: control of positioning of UDT catheters, bladder image during filling, trabeculation and diverticulae, VUR, urethral outflow obstruction as with DSD, inflow of contrast solution in the prostate, cystocele/urethrocele, urethral diverticulae, calculi, and more.

5.9   One Channel UDT

The equipment needed is an infusing stand, a bottle with sterile infusion liquid (NaCl 0.9%, 500 ml) connected with a three-way connector or Y-tube (Fig. 5.1). The channel I is connected to a Nelaton catheter (FR 12–14) introduced transurethrally into the bladder. The channel II is connected with a glass (less frequently used) or plastic tube with open top, fixed against a one-meter measure, with divisions of 1 cm, put vertically against the stand. This is used for Pves measurement. The channel III is connected with the filling tube. If the channel IV is needed for emptying the bladder between tests, it can be added through an extra Y valve to the three-way valve.

All tubes are filled with saline, and the zero of the pressure line is positioned at bladder level or pubic symphysis level. A collecting device is put at the meatal area (urinal, bed pan) for eventual voiding or leakage.

Filling rate is determined beforehand by opening the roller valve of the filling tube slowly and using a stop watch and volume flown out in a container. When filling rate remains stable, after being measured two to three times, the roller valve is fixed with a strip to make inflow fairly constant. The filling tube is clamped closer to the reservoir and filling will start when declamping is done. Patient is instructed to report bladder-filling sensations and other nonspecific symptoms that may occur.

Before starting, the liquid in the pressure tube, which has fallen to intravesical pressure, is controlled on rising with coughing. The start Pves is measured and together with start time noted on a special log sheet (Fig. 5.2). Infusion is started at the pre-set speed and the pressure noted every 30 s as presented in Fig. 5.2. The estimated filling volume is calculated from filling time x filling speed. Reported bladder-filling sensations and signs such as leakage, increased leg spasticity and signs of autonomic dysreflexia (such as rising of blood pressure) are recorded on the log sheet. The test is repeated after bladder emptying to check consistency. In case of voiding, post-void residual (PVR) volume is measured.

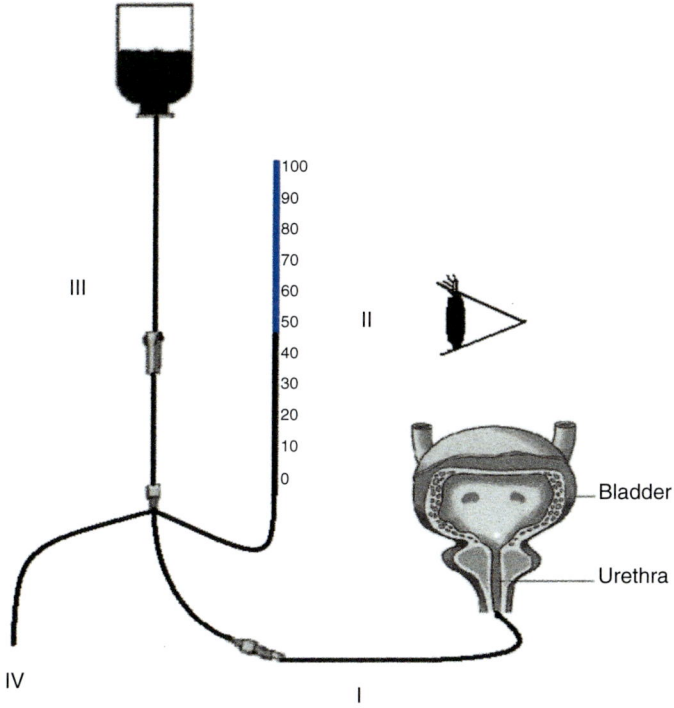

Fig. 5.1 One channel cystometry equipment. Channel I connected to bladder catheter; channel II for pressure measurement; channel III for filling the bladder; channel IV (eventually added) for bladder emptying (Wyndaele JJ, et al. Spinal Cord. 2009;47:526–30, with permission) [7]

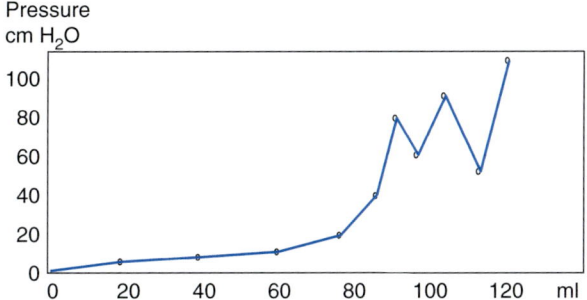

Fig. 5.2 Example of a log sheet with a tracing obtained with a one channel cystometry at 40 ml/min. Pressure development observed continuously. A patient is 48-year-old man with paraplegia T6, AIS-A, 12 weeks after injury. Cystometry shows NDO with high pressure development (Wyndaele JJ, et al. Spinal Cord. 2009;47:526–30, with permission) [7]

Sensation of filling can be defined as normal, increased (too strong, at small capacity), reduced (only one sensation—desire to void, or sensation only when the bladder is strongly filled), or as absent (as one of the signs of complete neurologic lesion).

Detrusor function during filling cystometry can be defined as normal with non-involuntary contraction during filling and no high pressure rise, as showing NDO or as detrusor areflexia.

Compliance is calculated (ml filling /cm H_2O pressure rise) between two standard points, which need to be determined: i.e. first point at start of filling, and second point just before the last involuntary detrusor contraction, or at first leakage, or at cystometric capacity, or at desire to void. Calculating between start and the maximum measured contraction pressure does not represent bladder compliance, as indication of expendability and related to bladder filling.

As even slow UDT filling rate is mostly above physiological diuresis, one can perform interrupted filling in consecutive steps, stopping infusion when pressure goes high and restarting when the pressure has dropped by adaptation of the wall (Fig. 6.1). This gives a more accurate estimation of pressure at higher filling volumes, and a more reliable compliance figure.

Normal detrusor function during voiding shows a voluntarily initiated continuous pressure rise, with evacuation of urine and complete bladder emptying. Such is rarely seen in neurogenic bladder after SCI, where often involuntary start of micturition is the case. The magnitude of the recorded pressure rise will give some indication of the degree of outlet resistance, or such resistance can be calculated electronically. Detrusor sphincter dyssynergia (DSD) can be suspected from the postponement of urine outflow despite high bladder-contraction pressure and by repeated interruption of the stream during voiding alternating with peaks of intravesical pressure.

In pressure-flow measurements, this can be more easily shown.

When available, Pura and/or EMG can help evaluate the sphincter activity during voiding.

J.J. Wyndaele, A. Kovindha, *Urodynamic Testing After Spinal Cord Injury*,
DOI 10.1007/978-3-319-54900-2_6

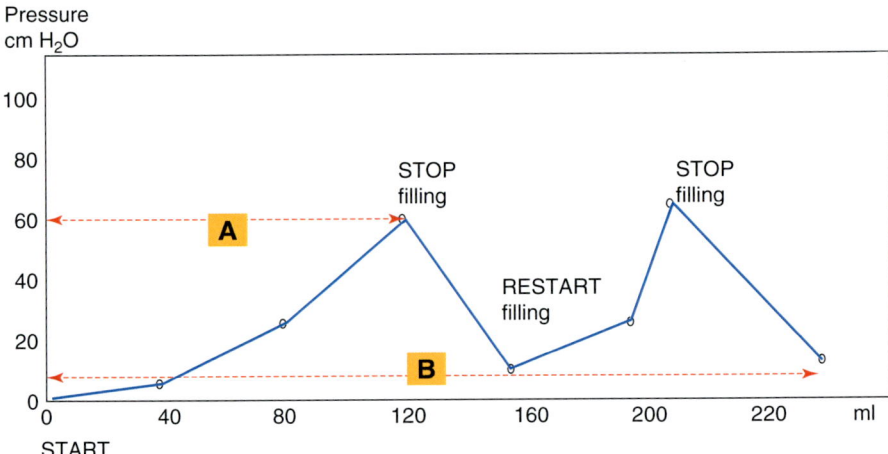

Fig. 6.1 Changes in measured bladder pressure showing differences in compliance calculation. Filling rate 100 ml/min. (*A*) Represents a wrong compliance calculation = 120/60 = 2 ml/cm H_2O. Pressure above 40 cm H_2O is obtained at 90 ml filling. When filling is stopped at higher pressure development, the pressure goes down again through adaptation of the bladder wall. (*B*) Represents a compliance calculation = 240/12 = 20 ml/cm H_2O

> Leak-point pressure, maximum vesical pressure during filling cystometry and cystometric bladder capacity are additional data obtained from UDT. Post-void residual (PVR) volume is measured when voiding is incomplete.

40 cm H$_2$O

Over the years, the development of a detrusor pressure above 40 cm H$_2$O has been accepted as dangerous for the upper urinary tract. Studies have shown deterioration of renal function and complication development in groups with cystometric pressure above 40 cm H$_2$O [9]. But some caution is needed. It still has to be evaluated how important the time is that pressure remains above 40 cm H$_2$O, if repeated high pressures from overactive contractions are as harmful as high pressure from low compliance, and how UDT tracings represent what happens in the LUT in daily life. Figure 7.1 gives some tracings of pressure change during cystometry. It is uncertain which is the most dangerous, though one may assume the danger C > B > A. This has however not been studied.

J.J. Wyndaele, A. Kovindha, *Urodynamic Testing After Spinal Cord Injury*, DOI 10.1007/978-3-319-54900-2_7

Detrusor pressure
cm H₂O

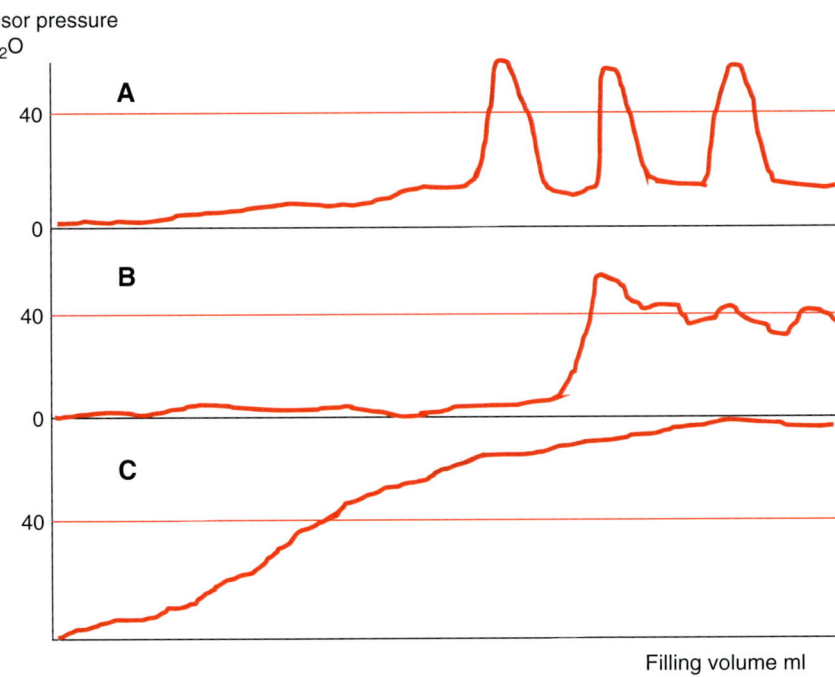

Fig. 7.1 Detrusor pressure development during UDT. A 40 cm H₂O pressure line is given. (*A*) Shows different short peaks of contraction pressure above the 40 cm line. (*B*) Shows sustained phasic detrusor contraction with pressure above 40 cm H₂O. (*C*) Shows a gradually rise of pressure from start of filling due to low bladder compliance

Training

8

Proper training is mandatory to permit the best clinical use of UDT. To perform the test, the experienced responsible physician can have trained allied professionals as UDT assistants. Interpretation is done by the physician and the UDT assistants together. To include the data from UDT in a comprehensive management, team discussion should be done, with conclusion on what is reliable, what is related to symptoms and signs, and which treatment should be given.

© Springer International Publishing AG 2017   27
J.J. Wyndaele, A. Kovindha, *Urodynamic Testing After Spinal Cord Injury*,
DOI 10.1007/978-3-319-54900-2_8

When to Perform UDT After SCI

9

There is no fixed time after SCI when the first UDT should be done. It depends on many factors: when patients are admitted, complications as UTI that need to be cured first, availability of UDT personnel, room and equipment. One should aim to get information after the period of spinal shock of the LUT, but it is not seldom uncertain when this period has ended.

Mostly the first UDT is done on average at 2 months after SCI. With very early transfer to the rehab unit and when neurological examination shows active sacral reflexes for suprasacral lesions or absence of such reflexes in cases of sacral/conal lesions, the first test, done at 4–6 weeks, can already provide important data. If, for one reason or another, the first UDT can only be performed at 4 or at 6 months post SCI, its clinical value is still high.

© Springer International Publishing AG 2017   29
J.J. Wyndaele, A. Kovindha, *Urodynamic Testing After Spinal Cord Injury*,
DOI 10.1007/978-3-319-54900-2_9

When to Repeat UDT

10

If the UDT shows that spinal shock is still present in supraspinal lesions, a new test can be scheduled 6 weeks to 2 months later. The UDT can be repeated if the first test is inconclusive, outcome of urological management not successful (refractory incontinence, complications, retention), or even as a routine evaluation after 4–6 months. If treatment has been started or changed, a control UDT, to evaluate the treatment effect, can be scheduled some weeks later, when the effect of the changes would probably be visible.

During follow-up after discharge, a yearly UDT is not advocated. In the long-term, the UDT tests done every 2–3 years in a symptom free SCI individual would permit to follow the urodynamic function well, but is not often performed due to practical reasons, the fear of complications or the lack of clinical value.

Children form a special group. They will have regular changes in the urodynamic situation when growing up. They need UDT at regular interval (yearly, and certainly at specific moments as when puberty starts, when they grow into adulthood).

© Springer International Publishing AG 2017   31
J.J. Wyndaele, A. Kovindha, *Urodynamic Testing After Spinal Cord Injury*,
DOI 10.1007/978-3-319-54900-2_10

Complications of UDT

11

Complications should be prevented by applying proper techniques and strictly following UDT rules, such as haematuria, oedema of the urinary bladder wall, bladder spasm, urethral trauma, autonomic dysreflexia attack have been reported, as well as bladder over-distension when the filling is continued too long.

The risk for symptomatic urinary tract infection (UTI) warrants antibiotic prophylaxis when UDT is done.

J.J. Wyndaele, A. Kovindha, *Urodynamic Testing After Spinal Cord Injury*,
DOI 10.1007/978-3-319-54900-2_11

Indications to Postpone UDT

12

UDT should be postponed when there is UTI, when macroscopic haematuria is seen, when autonomic dysreflexia (AD) prevention is not given in a patient with AD risk, when urethral pathology/sphincter spasticity prevents normal insertion of the bladder catheter. If a patient does not completely complies or agrees with performing the UDT, one should consider either postponing or declining it.

© Springer International Publishing AG 2017   35
J.J. Wyndaele, A. Kovindha, *Urodynamic Testing After Spinal Cord Injury*,
DOI 10.1007/978-3-319-54900-2_12

Special UDT Tests

13

Some special tests, such as ice water test or bethanechol super sensitivity test, have fallen in disuse, though they may have clinical value as reported demonstrated in literature.

13.1 Ice Water Test

The Ice water test (IWT) is based on the principle that introducing cold water (4°) into the bladder can elicit a spinal reflex contraction of the detrusor when inhibition by supraspinal centres is disturbed, as with SCI.

Originally described as bedside technique, a simultaneous measurement of intravesical pressure permits to rule out false negative tests. A positive test has been shown in 95% of patients with complete and 91% of those with incomplete suprasacral lesion. All patients with LUT denervation had a negative IWT [8–9]. Repeating the IWT has been shown to increase its positivity [10]. After sphinal shock, watch out for autonomic dysreflexia (AD) in those with spinal cord lesion at or above T6.

13.2 Bethanechol Super Sensitivity Test

This test was developed to distinguish between a neurologic and a myogenic aetiology of hypocontractile detrusor. Positive results have been described in neurologic and non-neurologic detrusor areflexia with sensitivity of 90%, and specificity of 95.6% [11]. Literature cautions on many variables which influence the outcome of the test. Application should be only subcutaneous. Strong general reactions due to excess parasympathetic stimulation has been described.

© Springer International Publishing AG 2017   37
J.J. Wyndaele, A. Kovindha, *Urodynamic Testing After Spinal Cord Injury*,
DOI 10.1007/978-3-319-54900-2_13

13.3   Clinical Neurophysiological Tests

Several clinical neurophysiologic tests have been used in research but have a limited role in routine diagnostics for SCI patients.

Evaluation of LUT afferent innervation can be done *with measurements of LUT electrical thresholds.* This specific semi-objective information is not otherwise obtainable. The test can be done during UDT but needs special equipment which is not cheap. Its main purpose is to evaluate if sensory nerves of the LUT have been intact which can transport filling sensation and desire to void to the brain. A positive test changes the diagnosis of those considered as AIS A or complete to incomplete lesion [12].

Rules to Get Proper Results of UDT

14

- Prepare equipment well, including correct calibration
- Perform a sterile technique of catheterization when handling the pressure and filling tubes
- Defaecation or bowel evacuation should be done the night before the UDT
- Use slow filling rate, preferably 10–30 ml/min. If a faster filling rate is used, take this into account when interpreting the results (as compliance, volume at first NDO contraction)
- Keep a continuous observation on what happens on the urodynamic tracings and with the patient
- Check regularly (by cough/pressure at abdomen) whether all catheters have remained in the correct position and continue to measure correctly
- Ask the patient to report sensations elicited by the filling, and every symptoms related to the UDT and symptoms of AD
- Administer antibacterial prophylaxis because there is a clear risk of UTI

© Springer International Publishing AG 2017
J.J. Wyndaele, A. Kovindha, *Urodynamic Testing After Spinal Cord Injury*,
DOI 10.1007/978-3-319-54900-2_14

Value of UDT

15

The UDT should be performed to find answers for the following questions:

- How is the urodynamic situation, cystometric capacity, detrusor pressure development?
- Is the emptying technique used appropriate and safe?
- Why does incontinence, recurrent infection, trabeculation/diverticula formation, autonomic dysreflexia develop?
- If video-urodynamics is used, is vesicoureteral reflux or other pathology in the LUT found? Is the bladder neck closed during filling and open during voiding?

© Springer International Publishing AG 2017

J.J. Wyndaele, A. Kovindha, *Urodynamic Testing After Spinal Cord Injury*,
DOI 10.1007/978-3-319-54900-2_15

Different Types of Intravesical Pressure Development

16

Several types of intravesical pressure development can be seen during filling UDT. The vesical pressure (Pves) tracings from a one channel cystometry are similar with the detrusor pressure (Pdet) tracings if correctly measured with a multi-channel UDT.

16.1 Three Types of Vesical Pressure Tracings from a One Channel Cystometry

Following are three examples from a one channel cystometry (Figs. 16.1, 16.2, and 16.3).

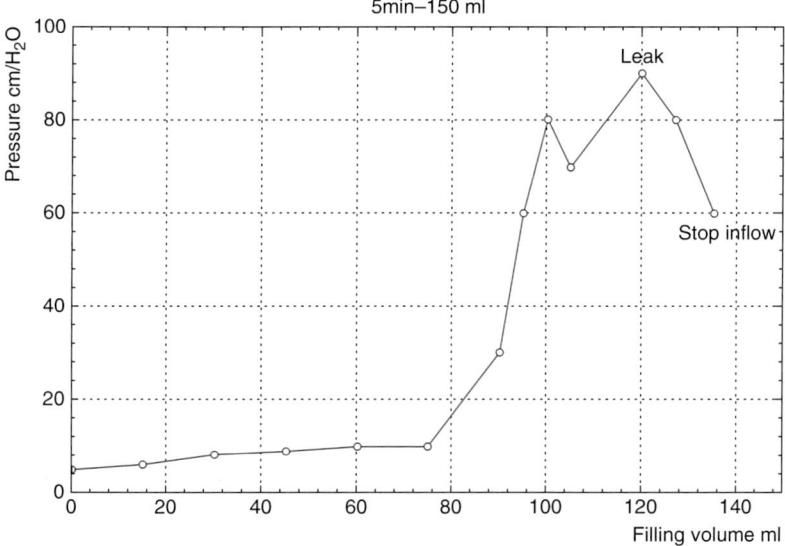

Fig. 16.1 Example of a volume-pressure tracing obtained from a one channel cystometry of a 22-year-old man with paraplegia T7, AIS A, 6 weeks after injury. It shows NDO, with high pressure (90 cm H_2O) leakage at volume of 120 ml (Wyndaele JJ, et al. Spinal Cord. 2009;47:526–30, with permission) [7]

© Springer International Publishing AG 2017
J.J. Wyndaele, A. Kovindha, *Urodynamic Testing After Spinal Cord Injury*,
DOI 10.1007/978-3-319-54900-2_16

43

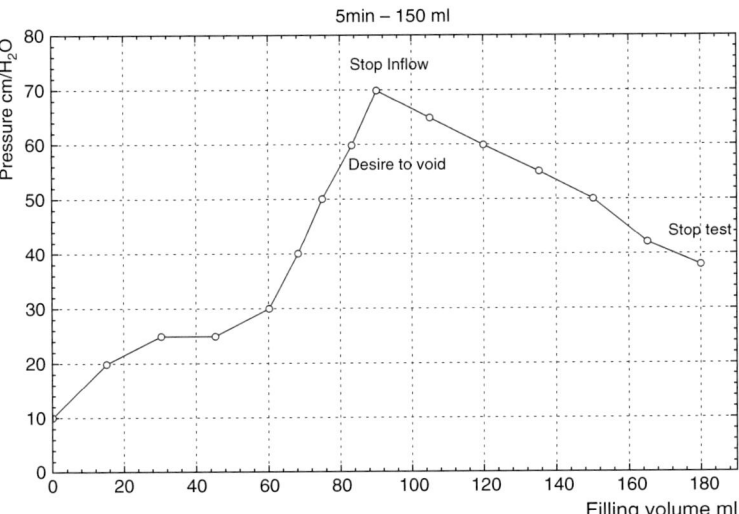

Fig. 16.2 Cystometry of a 32-year-old man with paraplegia T5, AIS-B, 6 months after SCI. Treatment with indwelling catheter for 6 months. Low bladder compliance is seen with high pressure development at low volume. The start pressure is 10 cm H_2O. The filling is stopped after pressure slowly rose and desire to void developed. Gradually the pressure has come down to 38 cm H_2O after stopping the inflow without leakage, indicating that the pressure rise is mainly due to loss of extensibility of the bladder wall = low compliance. Calculated compliance on this tracing from start to stop = 180 ml/28 cm H_2O = 6.2 ml/cm H_2O. (Wyndaele JJ, et al. Spinal Cord. 2009;47:526–30, with permission) [7]

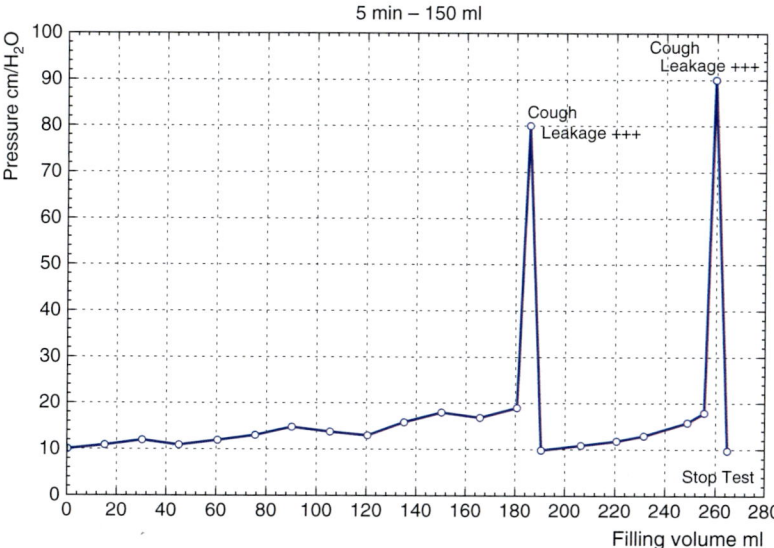

Fig. 16.3 Cystometry of a 57-year-old woman with paraplegia L1, AIS-A, 3 months after SCI. Leakage despite self-catheterization. The start pressure is 10 cm H_2O. Stress urinary incontinence demonstrated without bladder contraction. Cough leak point pressure $80-10 = 70$ cm H_2O. From start to stop no pressure difference is seen, indicating a high compliance. (Wyndaele JJ, et al. Spinal Cord. 2009;47:526–30, with permission) [7]

16.2   Advantage of Simultaneous Pressure Measurements in Bladder and Bowel

When bladder and rectal pressure tubes are available, and the detrusor pressure (Pdet) is calculated automatically, interpretation of intravesical pressure (Pves) rise often becomes more easy.

It is mandatory to look at all available tracings simultaneously to avoid pitfalls or misinterpretation (Figs. 16.4, 16.5, 16.6, and 16.7).

Fig. 16.4 Simultaneous measurement of Pves and Pabd, and calculation of the detrusor pressure (Pdet). Same pressure rise in bladder and in rectum shows an extravesical/intra-abdominal cause of the pressure rise, but no true bladder activity resulting in a flat Pdet tracing

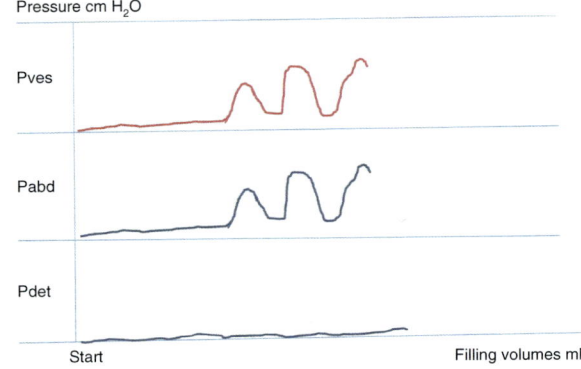

Fig. 16.5 Simultaneous measurement of Pves and Pabd, and calculation of Pdet. There is only pressure rise in the bladder pressure (Pves) tracing, and not in the rectal (Pabd) tracing. This indicates contractions of the bladder wall itself (see the Pdet tracing)

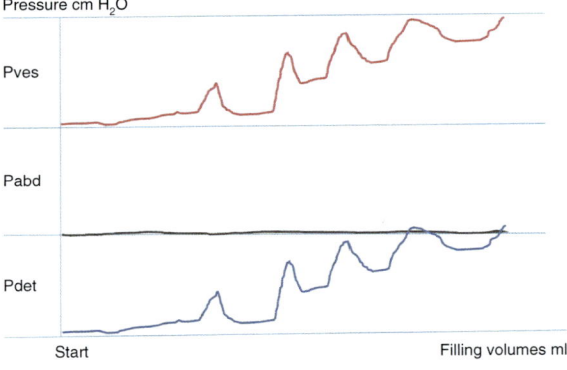

Fig. 16.6 Simultaneous measurement of Pves and Pabd, and calculation of Pdet. The slow pressure rise in Pves and Pdet but not in Pabd may indicate low bladder compliance. When the filling is stopped, the pressure adapts slowly. Restarting the filling creates again gradual pressure rise indicating low compliance. See also Fig. 16.2

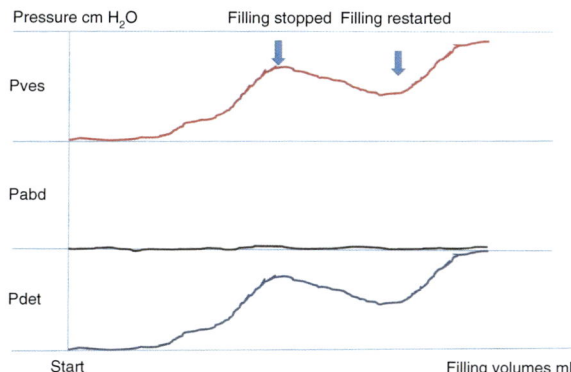

Fig. 16.7 Simultaneous measurement of Pves and Pabd, and calculation of Pdet. There is no pressure change in Pves but strong changes in the Pabd tracing, indicating bowel contractions. This causes negative deviations in the Pdet tracing.
Intraabdominal causes of pressure peaks are unlikely as they would be present on Pves tracing

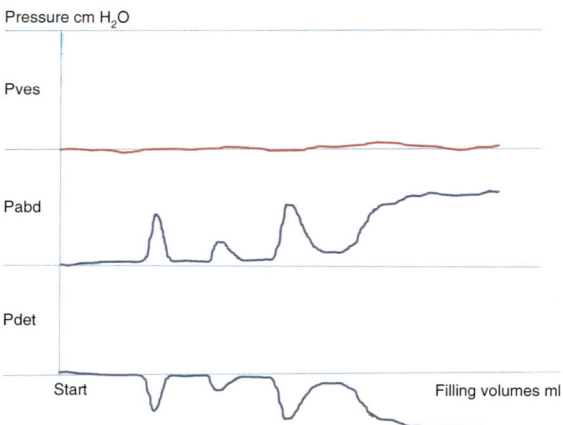

16.3   Adding a Urethral Sphincter Tracing

Sphincter function can be evaluated with EMG activity (Figs. 16.8 and 16.9), or with an intraurethral pressure catheter with openings at the level of the external sphincter (Figs. 17.1, 17.2, and 17.3). Most important is the diagnosis of detrusor sphincter dyssynergia (DSD). An example is given in Fig. 16.8.

In a normal person, the EMG activity also gradually increases with increasing volume in the bladder. During voiding the EMG shows relaxation of the sphincter.

Fig. 16.8 Four tracings of Pves, Pabd, Pdet and EMG of the urethral sphincter are followed together. During contractions of the bladder a simultaneous increase of the EMG signal (DSD) is seen preventing outflow of urine and adding to a further increase of the intravesical pressure

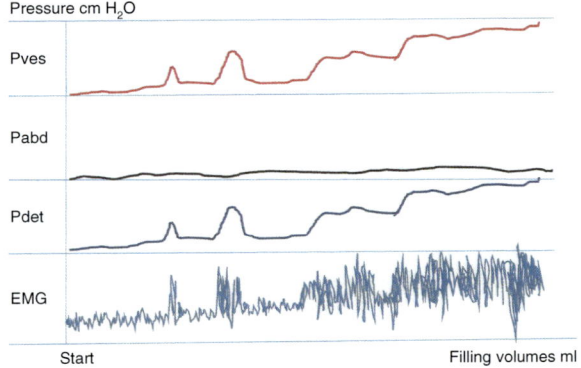

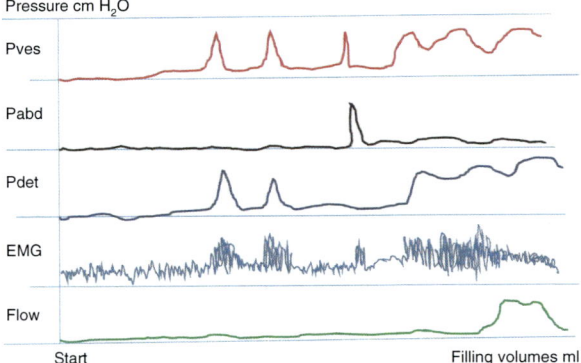

Fig. 16.9 Five tracings UDT of a SCI case shows NDO and finally leakage/incontinence. Two periods of overactive detrusor contractions are simultaneous with increased EMG activity. A cough gives the next pressure and EMG rise. Outflow from a more continuous overactive contraction is blocked by an initial increase in EMG activity. But as the detrusor contraction continues the urethral sphincter gets exhausted and relaxes, and urine outflow starts

16.4   Adding Uroflowmetry

Outflow of urine, including leakage, can be measured with a uroflowmetry. More information becomes available. An example of a 5 tracing UDT (Pves, Pabd, Pdet, EMG, Flow) is given in Fig. 16.9.

Urodynamic Tracings with Full Medical Files

17

17.1 Case 1

Figures 17.1 and 17.2

17.1.1 History

A 18 years old man.

Operated for tumor pinealis, radiotherapy, development of tethered cord, neurosurgical procedure 6 months ago. Voiding with Valsalva was changed to CISC 2 months ago. Constipation. Problems of ejaculation and erection.

17.1.1.1 LUT Function Basic Data Set

Urinary tract impairment unrelated to spinal cord injury: No

Awareness of the need to empty the bladder: Rarely desire to void and very rarely sensation of urgency mostly with leakage of small amount of urine.

Bladder emptying: Straining (abdominal straining, Valsalva's manoeuvre) 2 times a day, intermittent catheterization 2 times a day

Average number of voluntary bladder-emptyings per day during the last week: 4–5

Any involuntary urine leakage (incontinence) within the last three months: Yes

Collecting appliances for urinary incontinence: No

Any drugs for the urinary tract within the last year: Prophylaxis with nitrofurantoin daily

Surgical procedures on the urinary tract: No

Any change in urinary symptoms within the last year: Not applicable

© Springer International Publishing AG 2017
J.J. Wyndaele, A. Kovindha, *Urodynamic Testing After Spinal Cord Injury*,
DOI 10.1007/978-3-319-54900-2_17

17.1.2 Clinical Examination

Perineal sensation for touch: present
Cremaster reflex: + bilaterally
Anal sphincter tone: weak
No anal reflex, no bulbocavernosus reflex. No voluntary contraction of pelvic muscles.

17.1.3 Urodynamic Basic Data Set (see Fig. 17.1)

Bladder sensation during filling Radiography or Cystogram: Slight pressure
sensation at higher filling grade
Detrusor function: Neurogenic detrusor overactivity
Compliance during filling cystometry: Low= 10.2 mL/cm H_2O
Urethral Function during voiding: Spasticity, detrusor sphincter dyssynergia
(DSD) with relaxation during second contraction, 22 ml leakage

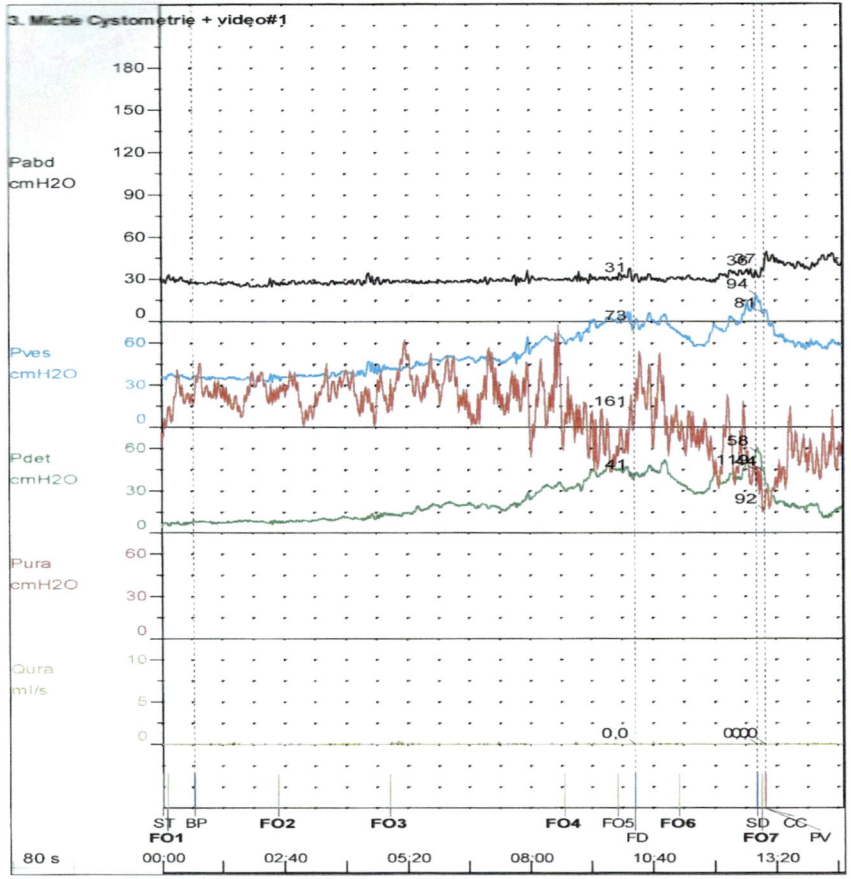

Fig. 17.1 Pdet at start is +8 cm H_2O. Little change in abdominal pressure. Pressure rises several
time in Pves and Pdet. Urethral tracing shows strong changes in pressure (spasticity). Minimal leakage. Detrusor zero line is not correct: detrusor pressure should be calculated −8 cm H_2O

Maximum detrusor pressure: _____50_____ cm H_2O
Cystometric bladder capacity: ___391_____ mL
Post void residual volume: ___369_____mL

17.1.4 Urinary Tract Imaging Basic Data Set (see Fig. 17.2)

Ultrasound of the urinary tract: Normal
X-ray of the urinary tract—Kidney Ureter Bladder: Normal (as seen in the first picture of the video-urodynamics, Fig. 7.2)
Renography: Not done
Bladder neck at rest: Open
Other findings: Image of trabeculated wall of bladder during filling. Contrast solution fills the posterior urethra from the start of filling indicating incompetent bladder neck

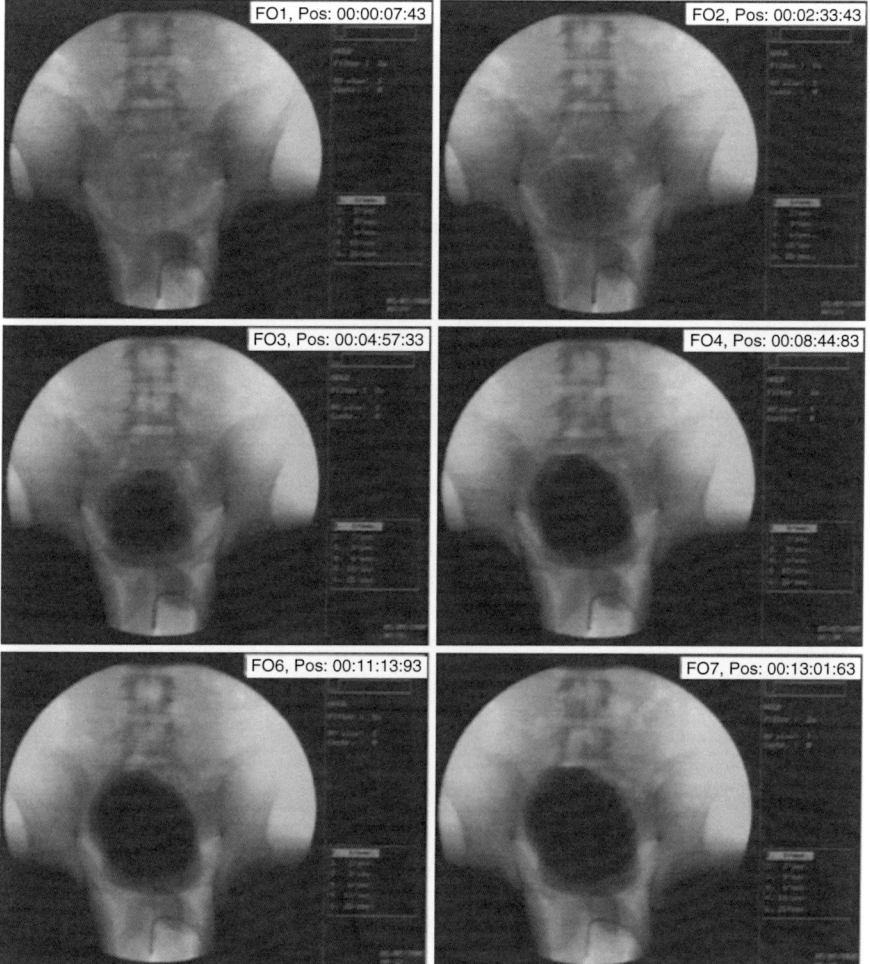

Fig. 17.2 Cystogram during video-urodynamic test shows open bladder neck and inflow contrast medium in the posterior urethra. FO numbers give sequence pictures taken

17.1.5 Other Diagnostic Tests

Cystoscopy: Bladder trabeculated, bladder neck widely open.
Electrodiagnostic tests: SSEP from penile stimulation shows no reproducible signals. EMG bulbocavernosus muscle shows denervation. Slow reflex latency of lumbosacral reflexes
Electrosensation bladder and urethra: High threshold but sensation is present

17.1.6 Management

Stop straining for voiding and perform CISC 4–5 per day. Antimuscarinic drug. UDT control in 4 months

17.2   Case 2

Figures 17.3 and 17.4

17.2.1 History

A 20 years old man, road traffic accident one year ago. T4 paraplegia, AIS A

17.2.1.1   LUT Function Basic Data Set
Urinary tract impairment unrelated to spinal cord injury: No
Awareness of the need to empty the bladder: No
Bladder emptying: Intermittent self-catheterization
Average number of voluntary bladder emptying per day during the last week: 6
Any involuntary urine leakage (incontinence) within the last three months: Very frequent leakage
Collecting appliances for urinary incontinence: Condom catheter
Any drugs for the urinary tract within the last year: Antimuscarinic
Surgical procedures on the urinary tract: No
Any change in urinary symptoms within the last year: No, clear urine
Other: Bowel: laxative 3/week, very rarely fecal incontinence. Reflex erection. UTI, now under antibiotics. Clear urine.

17.2.2 Clinical Examination

Perineal sensation for touch: positive left side; cremateric reflex: positive both sides. Tone anal sphincter: normal; anal reflex: positive, bulbocaversosus reflex: positive even with spasticity running into left lower limb. Contraction of pelvic muscles and anal sphincter: absent
   Small penile skin lesion from condom catheter

17.2.3 Urodynamic Basic Data Set (see Fig. 17.3)

Filling rate 30 ml/min
Bladder sensation during filling cystometry: Absent
Detrusor function: Detrusor overactivity at 50 ml bladder filling, high pressures, leakage.
Compliance during filling cystometry: 4 ml/cm H_2O
Urethral Function: Dyssynergic sphincter contraction during detrusor contraction
Maximum detrusor pressure: ___154_____ cm H_2O
Cystometric bladder capacity: ___60_____ mL
Post void residual volume: _____50___mL

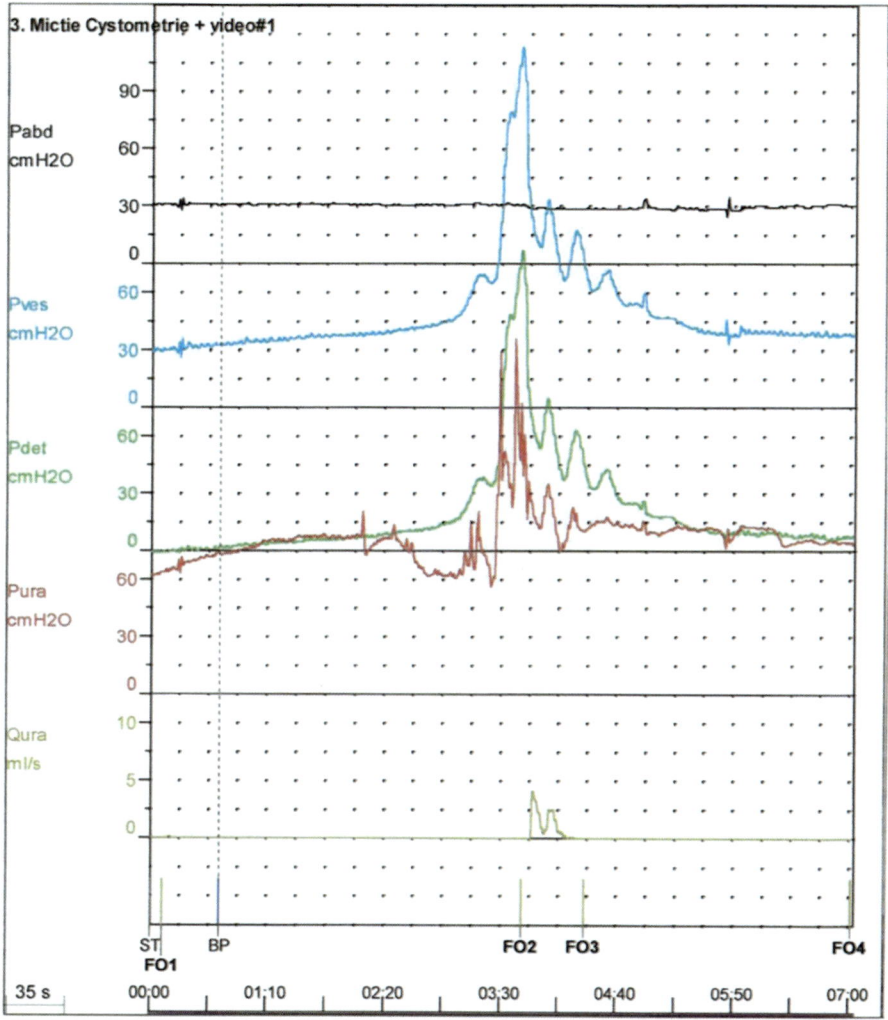

Fig. 17.3 Pdet at start is 0 cm H_2O. Filling rate 30 ml/min. No change in Pabd during filling. Pdet and Pves rise quickly indicating low compliance. High pressure overactive contractions and DSD. Involuntary micturition with incomplete bladder emptying

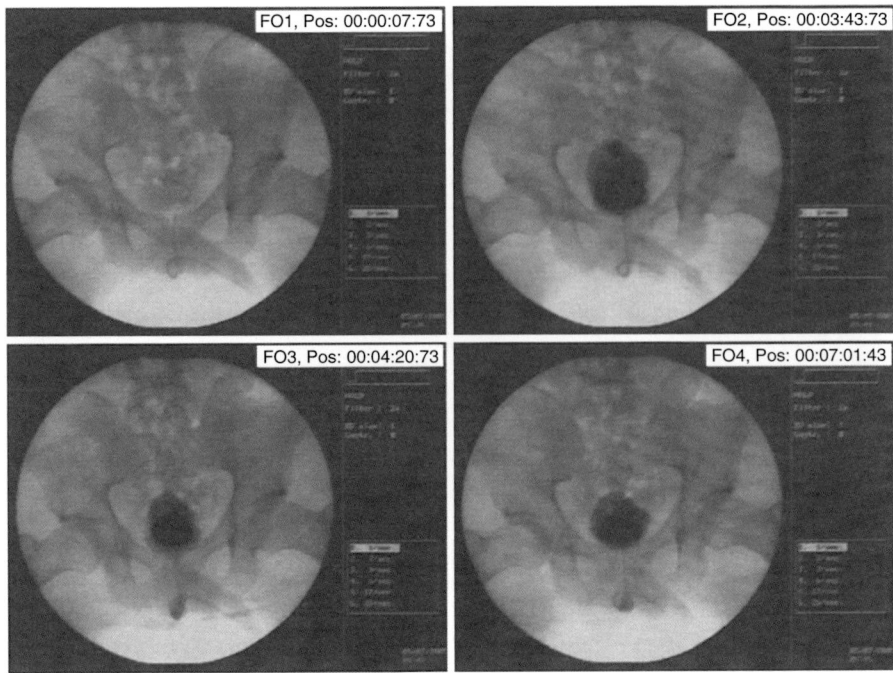

Fig. 17.4 Small trabeculated bladder. Flow into urethra posterior during involuntary voiding. Possibility grade 1 reflex right side but only visible very shortly on video during contraction of the bladder. FO numbers give sequences pictures taken

17.2.4 Urinary Tract Imaging Basic Data Set (see Fig. 17.4)

Ultrasound of the urinary tract: Stasis/dilatation in upper urinary tract, right side and left side
X-ray of the urinary tract—Kidney Ureter Bladder: Normal
Renography: Not done
Cystogram: Vesicoureteric reflux Right, closed bladder neck at rest
Video-urodynamic
Bladder neck during voiding: Normal
Vesicoureteric reflux: Absent
Striated urethral sphincter during voiding: Closed (dyssynergia)
Other findings: Small bladder, trabeculation, flow into urethra posterior during leakage. Possibility grade 1 reflex right side but only visible very shortly on video during contraction of the bladder.

17.2.5 Other Diagnostic Tests

Cystoscopy: Eggshell stones, trabeculation bladder wall
Electrosensation bladder and urethra: Perception of electrical current in bladder and urethra indicating passage through afferent nerve fibers towards the cortex
Special test: Ice water test 20 ml at 4 Celsius shows very strong contraction of bladder

Egg shell stones are often not visible on x-ray

17.2.6 Management

Lithotripsy of the stones.

Control urodynamic test after 3 weeks showed same high pressure contraction of the detrusor and dyssynergia. No UTI. Higher dose antimuscarinics and intermittent catheterization.

Result: No leakage, bladder capacity 250 ml. Compliance 12 ml/cm H_2O. NDO. Botulinum toxin injection resulted in good capacity, low pressure bladder with normal compliance.

17.3   Case 3

Figures 17.5, 17.6, and 17.7

17.3.1 History

A 30 years old man, road traffic accident two years ago. C7 tetraplegia, AIS C

17.3.1.1   LUT Function Basic Data Set
Urinary tract impairment unrelated to spinal cord injury: No
Awareness of the need to empty the bladder: Yes when full
Bladder emptying: Intermittent self catheterization
Average number of voluntary bladder emptyings per day during the last week: 4
Any involuntary urine leakage (incontinence) within the last three months: Very frequent leakage which disappeared under higher dosage of antimuscarinic drugs
Collecting appliances for urinary incontinence: No
Any drugs for the urinary tract within the last year: Antimuscarinic drugs, Oxybutinine 3×5 mg and changed to tolterodine retard 1/day
Surgical procedures on the urinary tract: No
Any change in urinary symptoms within the last year: Yes, 4 months ago autonomic dysreflexia, smaller bladder capacity, leakage. Higher dosage of oxybutynin made symptoms disappear but because of severe xerostomia it was changed to, tolterodine retard.
Other: After accident orthopaedic surgery with spondylodesis, interbody cage C5-C6, corporectomy C7, osteosynthese plate C6-T-2. Postoperatively rhabdomyolysis.

17.3.2 Clinical Examination

Urine: macroscopic clear, perianal sensation for touch: positive; cremasteric reflex positive: both sides, anal sphincter tone: normal; anal reflex: positive, bulbo reflex: positive. Voluntary contraction of pelvic muscles and anal sphincter: absent.

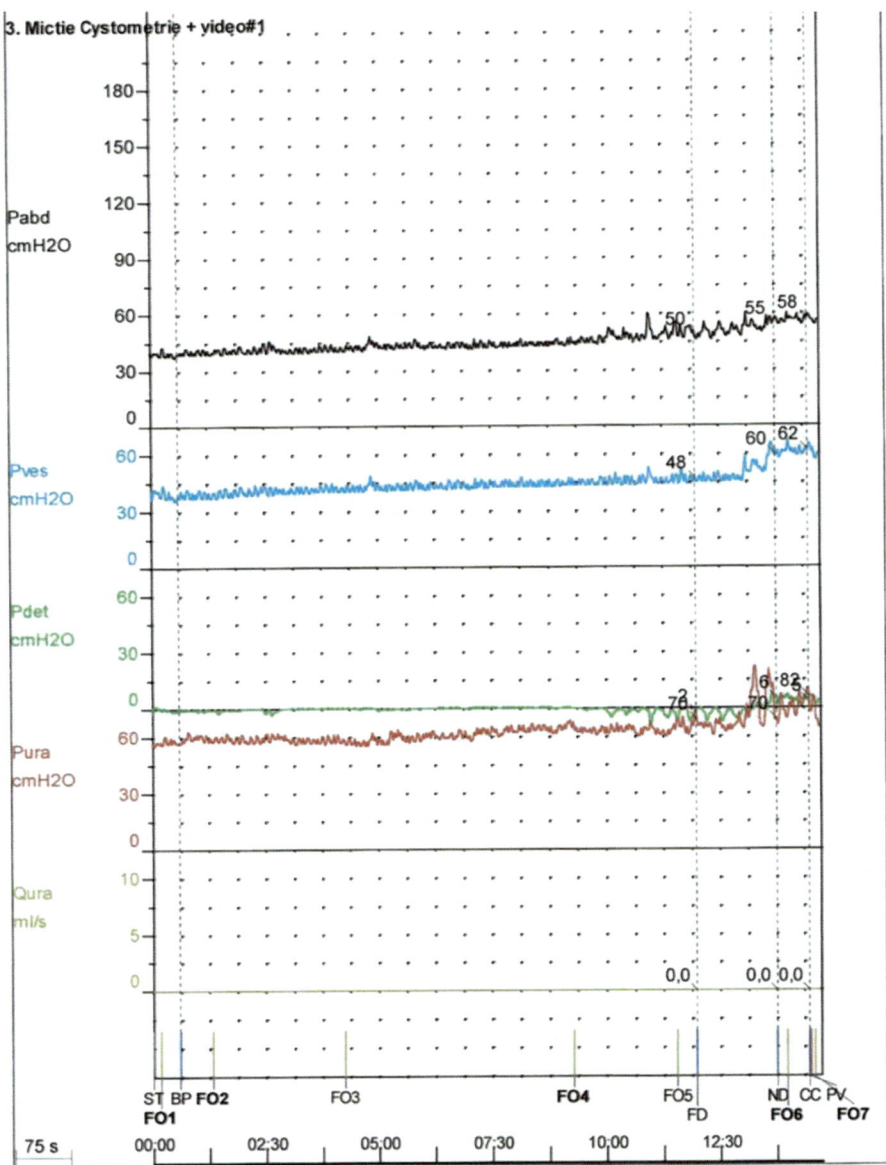

Fig. 17.5 Pdet at start is 0 cm H₂O. Filling rate 30 ml/min. Low Pabd rises at the end of bladder filling. No Pdet rise during filling indicates normal compliance. Low pressure NDO and DSD at end filling. FD = first sensation. ND = normal desire to void

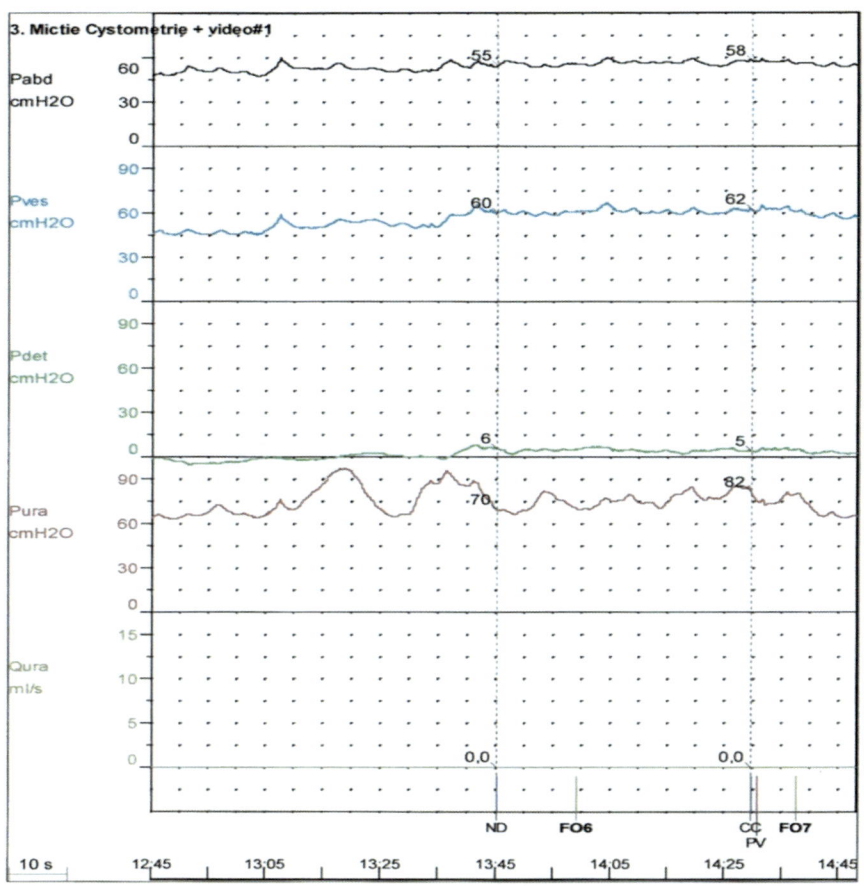

Fig. 17.6 Enlarged image of end of filling showing low pressure NDO and DSD

17.3.3 Urodynamic Basic Data Set (see Figs. 17.5 and Fig. 17.6)

Filling rate 30 ml/min.
Bladder sensation during filling cystometry: Feels filling of bladder: first sensation at 488 ml, sensation of desire to void at 567 ml.
Detrusor function: Low pressure NDO at 499 ml. No leakage
Compliance during filling cystometry: No Pdet rise from start filling to start of overactive contraction
Urethral Function: DSD
Maximum detrusor pressure: ___5_____ cm H2O
Cystometric bladder capacity: ___600_____ mL
Post void residual volume: _____Not applicable, no voiding___

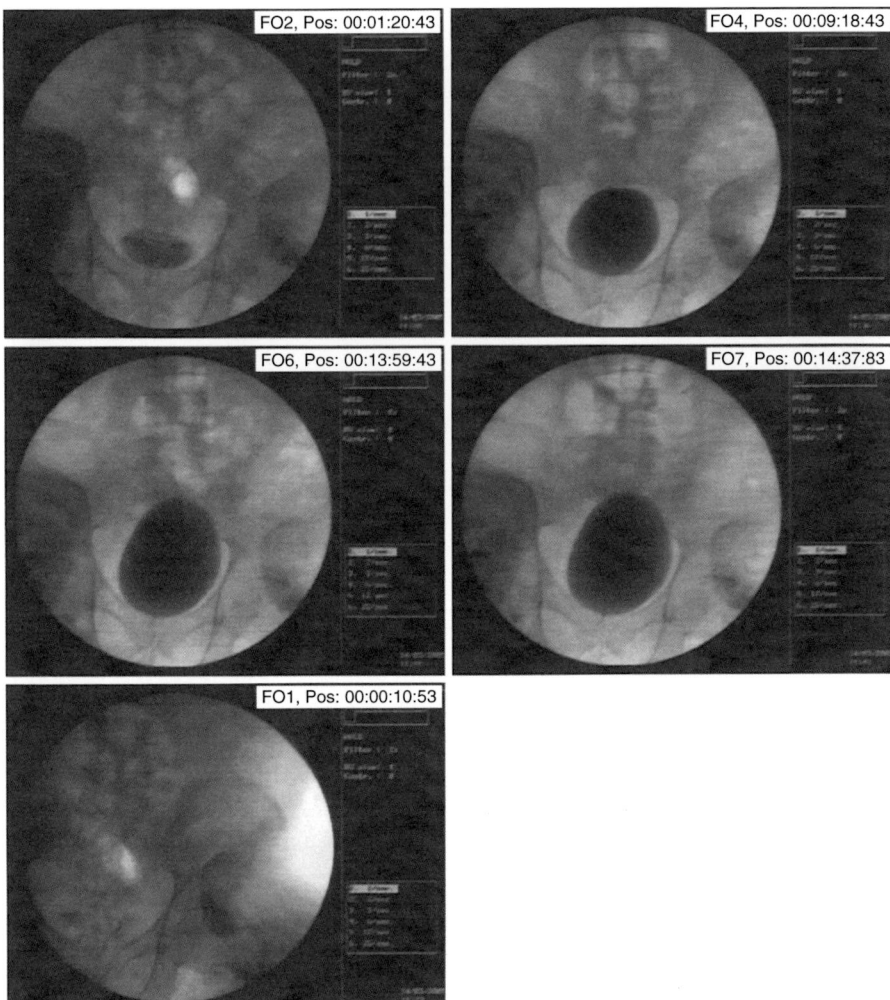

Fig. 17.7 During filling: normal image of bladder, bladder neck closed. No contrast in urethra. FO numbers = sequence pictures taken. Pictures not given in actual sequence

17.3.4 Urinary Tract Imaging Basic Data Set (see Fig. 17.7)

Ultrasound of the urinary tract: Normal
X-ray of the urinary tract – Kidney Ureter Bladder: Normal at start video-urodynamics
Renography: Not done
Cystogram: Normal
Voiding cystogram: No voiding

17.3.5 Other Diagnostic Tests

Cystoscopy: Not done
Electrosensation bladder and urethra: Higher threshold of perception of electrical current in bladder and urethra indicating passage through sensory nerve fibers towards the cortex

17.3.6 Management

CISC and antimuscarinics continued.

17.4   Case 4

Figures 17.8, 17.9, and 17.10

17.4.1 History

A 63 years old man, aortic dissection 1 year ago with paraplegia 9, AIS C

17.4.1.1   LUT Function Basic Data Set
Urinary tract impairment unrelated to spinal cord injury: No
Awareness of the need to empty the bladder: Yes
Bladder emptying: Voluntary voiding with high residual, involuntary voiding of large quantities, intermittent catheterization 3 times per week. Clear urine.
Average number of voluntary bladder-emptyings per day during the last week: 4
Any involuntary urine leakage (incontinence) within the last three months: very frequent leakage
Collecting appliances for urinary incontinence: Diaper
Any drugs for the urinary tract within the last year: No, but multiple drugs for blood pressure, kidney and heart
Surgical procedures on the urinary tract: No
Any change in urinary symptoms within the last year: No
Other: When aortic dissection happened he was urgently operated and a long period followed in critical care with priapism, fasciotomy left leg, hemodialysis during 3 weeks, suprapubic catheter, depression.

17.4.2 Clinical Examination

Perineal sensation for touch: absent; cremateric reflex: positive both sides. Tone anal sphincter: normal; anal reflex: positive, bulbocaversosus reflex: positive. Voluntary contraction pelvic muscles and anal sphincter: weak

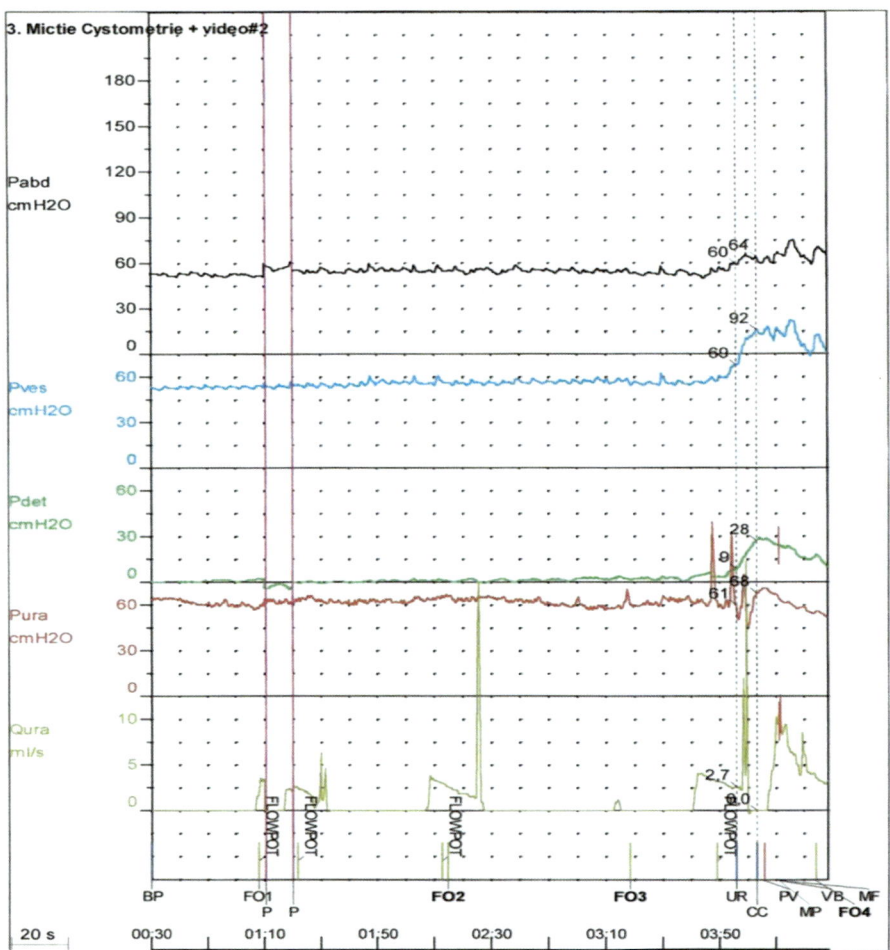

Fig. 17.8 Pdet at start is 0 cm H$_2$O. Filling rate 30 ml/min. Limited Pdet rise during filling indicating normal compliance. Involuntary start of voiding with DSD at start of bladder contraction followed by relaxation of the sphincter. Problems with Qura tracing due to partial blockage of disc in flowmeter. Only the last curve represents uroflow

17.4.3 Urodynamic Basic Data Set (see Figs. 17.8 and Fig. 17.9)

Filling rate 30 ml/min
Bladder sensation during filling cystometry: Sensation urgency at 193 ml
Detrusor function: Detrusor pressure 0 cm H$_2$O at start. NDO at 199 ml
Compliance during filling cystometry: 3 cm H$_2$O pressure rise from start to end filling (before NDO) = 199/3 = 66 ml/cm H$_2$O

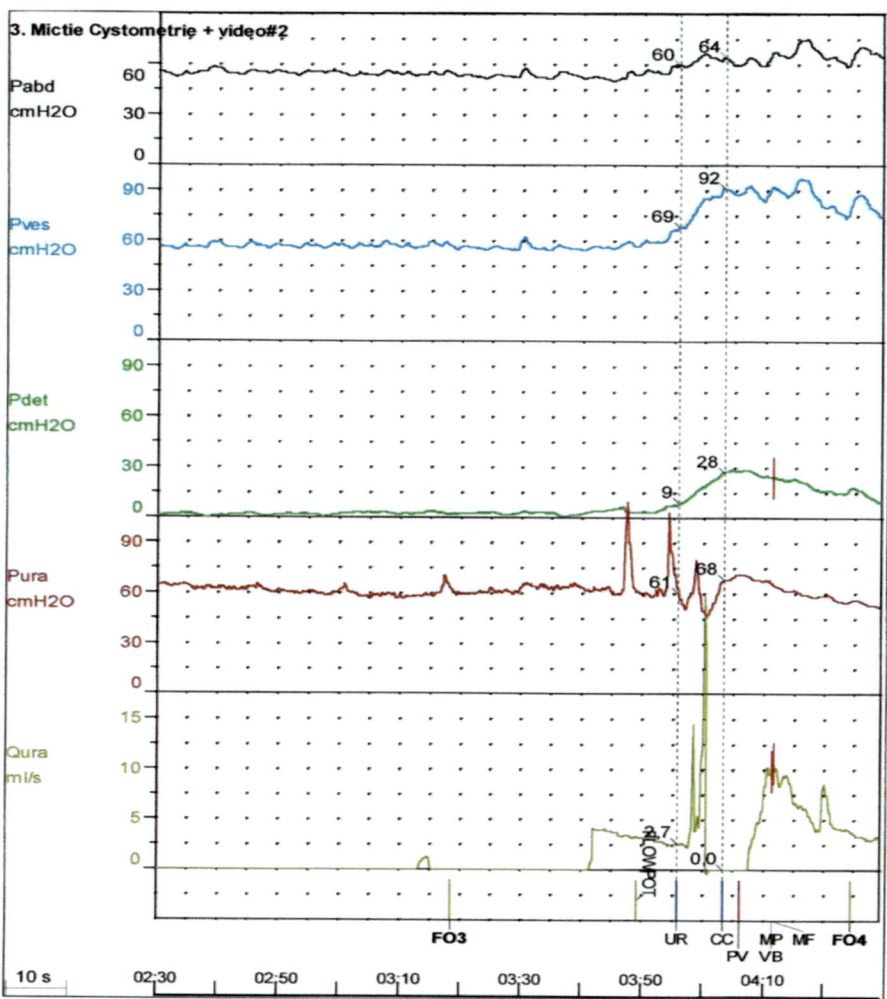

Fig. 17.9 Enlarged image of end of filling showing some pressure rise in Pabd. NDO with normal voiding pressure. DSD at start voiding only. Voiding with small residual. Technical problems with Qura tracing due to partial blockage of disc in uroflowmeter

Urethral Function: Contractions at start bladder contraction but relaxation afterwards with voiding

Maximum detrusor pressure: ___28_____ cm H_2O

Cystometric bladder capacity: ___199_____ mL

Post void residual volume: _____20 ml

Uroflow: Qmax 10.7 ml/s, average flow rate 5.5 ml/s, flow time 18 s, voiding time 18 s, time to qmax 0 s___

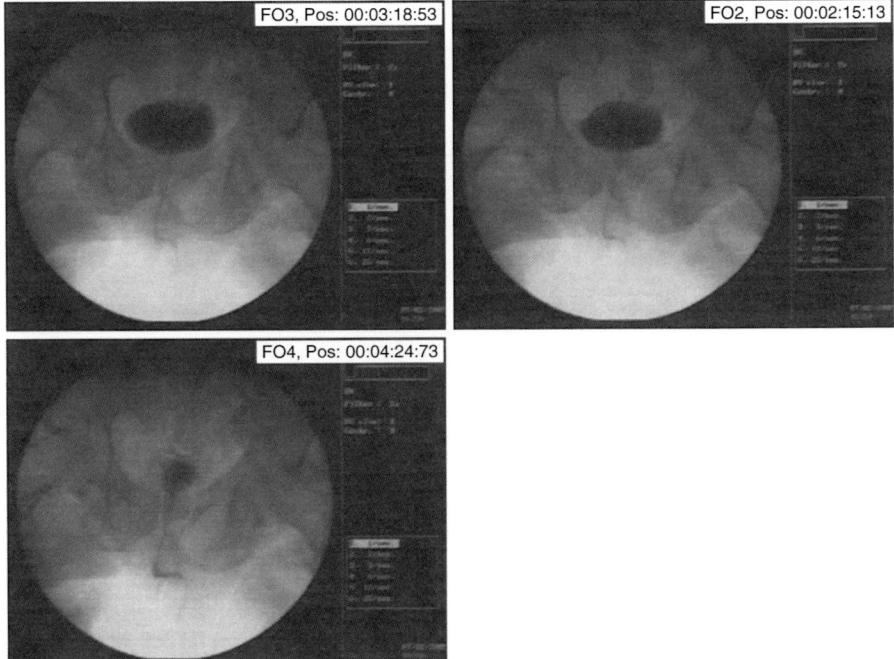

Fig. 17.10 Plain X-ray from start is missing. FO numbers give sequence of pictures taken. Normal image of bladder, bladder neck closed during filling. Voiding with normal passage through the urethra. Small residual urine not depicted here

17.4.4 Urinary Tract Imaging Basic Data Set (see Fig. 17.10)

Ultrasound of the urinary tract: Normal
X-ray of the urinary tract—Kidney Ureter Bladder: Normal at start videourodynamics (image not shown in Fig. 17.10)
Renography: Not done
Cystogram: Normal
Voiding cystogram: Normal

17.4.5 Other Diagnostic Tests

Cystoscopy: Not done
Electrosensation bladder and urethra: Perception of electrical current in bladder and urethra indicating passage through afferent nerve fibres to cortex, but higher threshold
Ice water test: Positive

17.4.6 Management

Teach CISC 4/day and start antimuscarinics. If leakage continues, increase dosage of antimuscarinics and cystoscopy to exclude local bladder pathology.

17.5   Case 5

Figures 17.11, 17.12, and 17.13

17.5.1 History

A 32 years old man, 3 months ago fell from height with T11 paraplegia, AIS B

17.5.1.1   LUT Function Basic Data Set
Urinary tract impairment unrelated to spinal cord injury: No
Awareness of the need to empty the bladder: No
Bladder emptying: CISC 4 per day with clear urine
Average number of voluntary bladder-emptying per day during the last week: 4
Any involuntary urine leakage (incontinence) within the last three months: Regularly leakage when making transfers
Collecting appliances for urinary incontinence: Diaper
Any drugs for the urinary tract within the last year: No
Surgical procedures on the urinary tract: No
Any change in urinary symptoms within the last year: Not applicable
Other: No erection, no sensation of defecation, manual evacuation of stool

17.5.2 Clinical Examination

Urine: Macroscopical clear. Perineal sensation for touch: negative. Cremasteric reflex: negative both sides. Anal sphincter tone: open sphincter; anal reflex: negative, bulbocavernosus reflex: negative. Voluntary contraction of pelvic muscles and anal sphincter: not possible

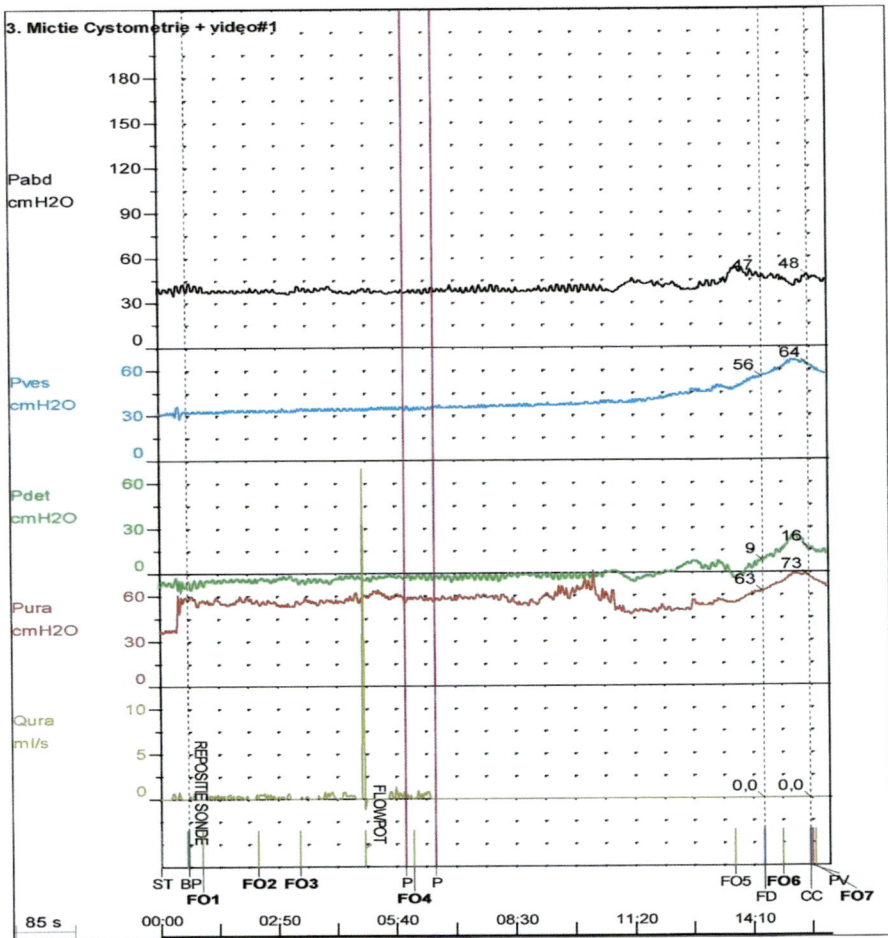

Fig. 17.11 Pdet at start is −4 cm H₂O. Filling rate 30 ml/min. Slow pressure rises at end bladder filling, normal compliance. Abdominal pressure undulates at end of filling giving undulating in Pdet tracing. FD = first desire to void = heaviness in lower abdomen. Artifacts in flow line during first part of cystometry because blocking in uroflowmeter

17.5.3 Urodynamic Basic Data Set (see Figs. 17.11 and 17.12)

Filling rate 30 ml/min

Bladder sensation during filling cystometry: Sensation of some heaviness in pelvic region at 597 ml. Does not increase when further filled up to 651 ml.

Detrusor function: Detrusor pressure −4 cm H₂O at start. Detrusor areflexia. Leakage when getting on the urodynamic table

Compliance during filling cystometry: 26 cm H₂O pressure rise from start to end filling. Calculated compliance 25.2 ml/cm H₂O

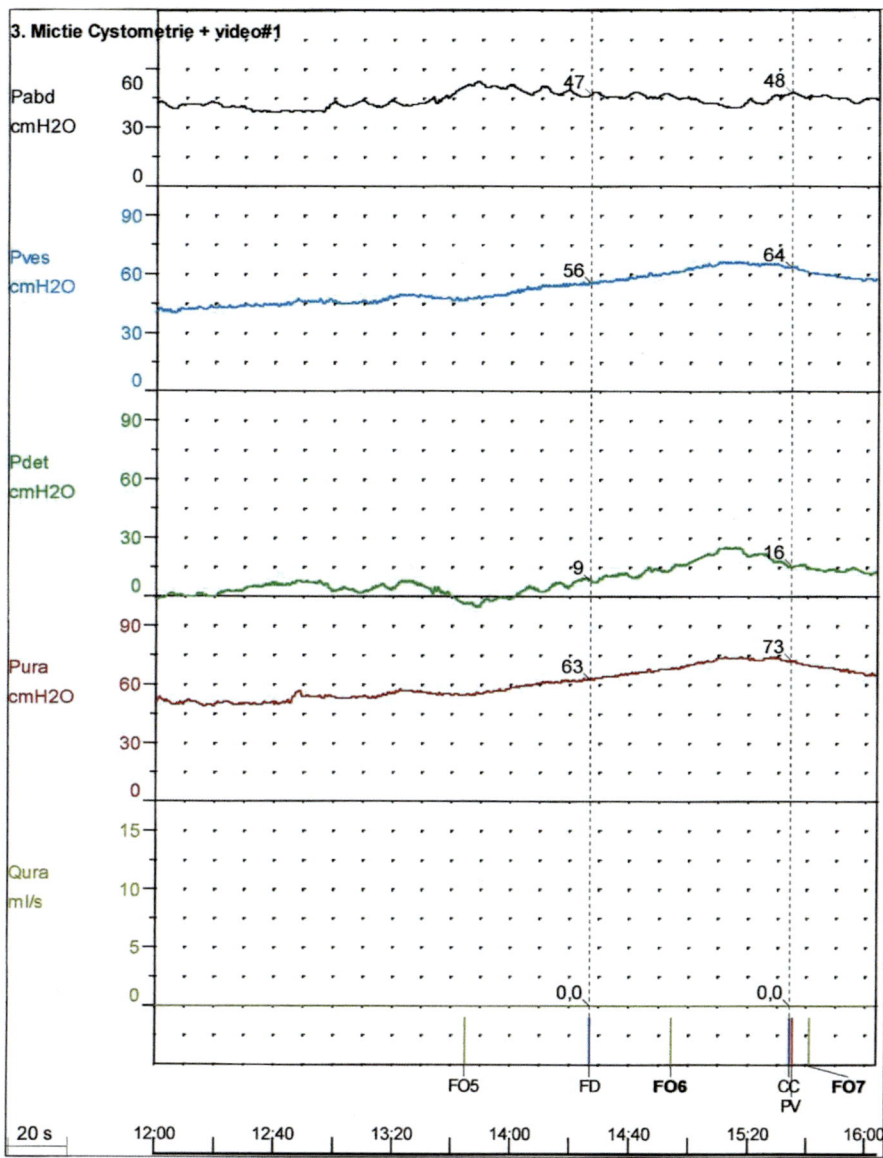

Fig. 17.12 Enlarged image of end of filling showing some pressure rise in Pves and Pdet. Ondulations in Pabd

Urethral Function: Little change in pressure during filling. Pressure rises at end of filling.
Maximum detrusor pressure: ___16 + 4 = 20_____ cm H$_2$O
Cystometric bladder capacity: ___651_____ mL
Post void residual volume: _____651 ml
Uroflow: no flow.

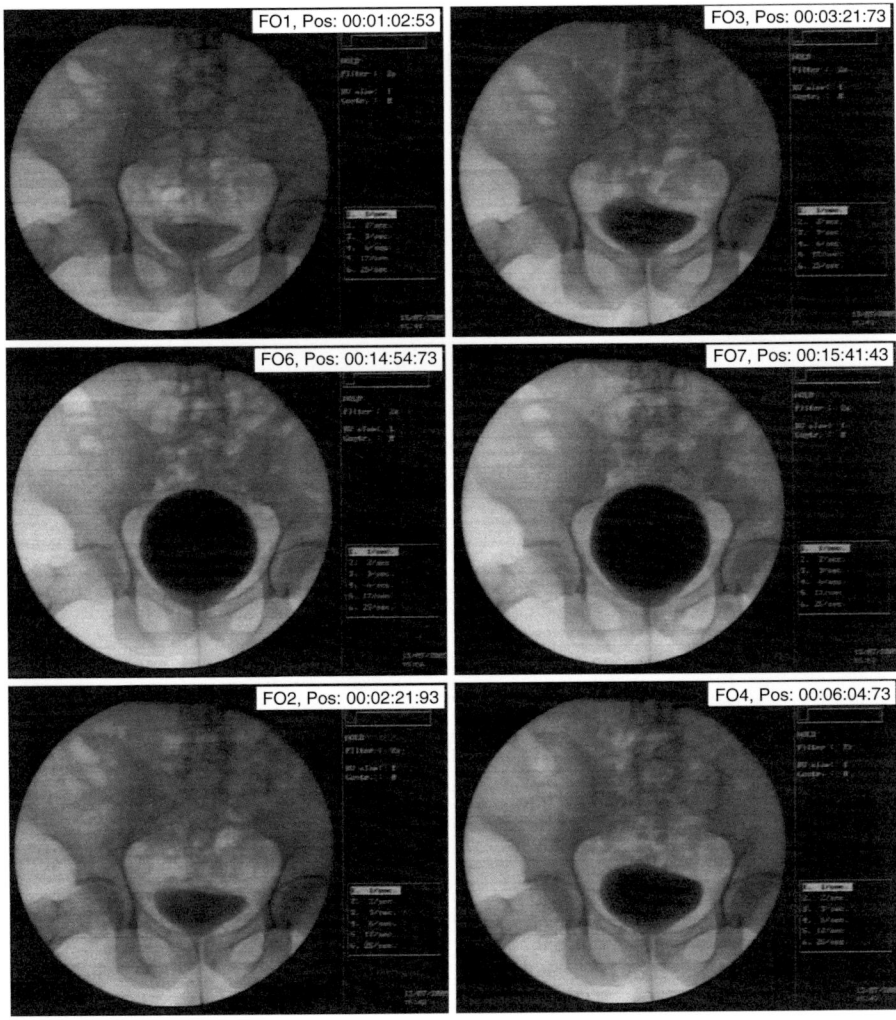

Fig. 17.13 Normal image of bladder. Bladder neck opens with some contrast solution leaking in the prostatic urethra. FO number gives sequence of pictures taken

17.5.4 Urinary Tract Imaging Basic Data Set (see Fig. 17.13)

Ultrasound of the urinary tract: Normal
X-ray of the urinary tract—Kidney Ureter Bladder: Normal at start of video-urodynamics (not depicted in Fig. 17.13)
Renography: Not done
Cystogram: Bladder neck opens at rest
Other findings: Normal bladder, with open bladder neck and inflow of contrast in proximal urethra during filling
Voiding cystogram: No voiding

17.5.5 Other Diagnostic Tests

Cystoscopy: Not done
Electrosensation bladder and urethra: Not done

17.5.6 Management

CISC.
  Because of bothersome leakage implantation of artificial sphincter AS800 around bladder neck. Not completely dry but very much improved.

17.6   Case 6

Figures 17.14, 17.15, and 17.16

17.6.1 History

A 47 years old woman, road traffic accident 16 months ago, T8 paraplegia, AIS A

17.6.1.1   LUT Function Basic Data Set
Urinary tract impairment unrelated to spinal cord injury: No
Awareness of the need to empty the bladder: No
Bladder emptying: Suprapubic catheter because of body weight and personal choice, clear urine
Average number of voluntary bladder emptyings per day during the last week: Not applicable
Any involuntary urine leakage (incontinence) within the last three months: Rarely leakage beside catheter
Collecting appliances for urinary incontinence: Diaper
Any drugs for the urinary tract within the last year: Botulinum toxin in detrusor 8 months ago
Surgical procedures on the urinary tract: Botulinum toxin injcetion
Any change in urinary symptoms within the last year: No

17.6.2 Clinical Examination

Urine: macroscopic clear, perineal sensation for touch: negative. Anal sphincter tone: normal; anal reflex: positive, bulbocavernosus reflex: positive. Voluntary contraction of pelvic muscles and anal sphincter: absent

17.6.3 Urodynamic Basic Data Set (see Figs. 17.14 and 17.15)

Filling rate 30 ml/min
Bladder sensation during filling cystometry: Sensation of filling at 474 ml
Detrusor function: Pdet = 0 cm H_2O at start

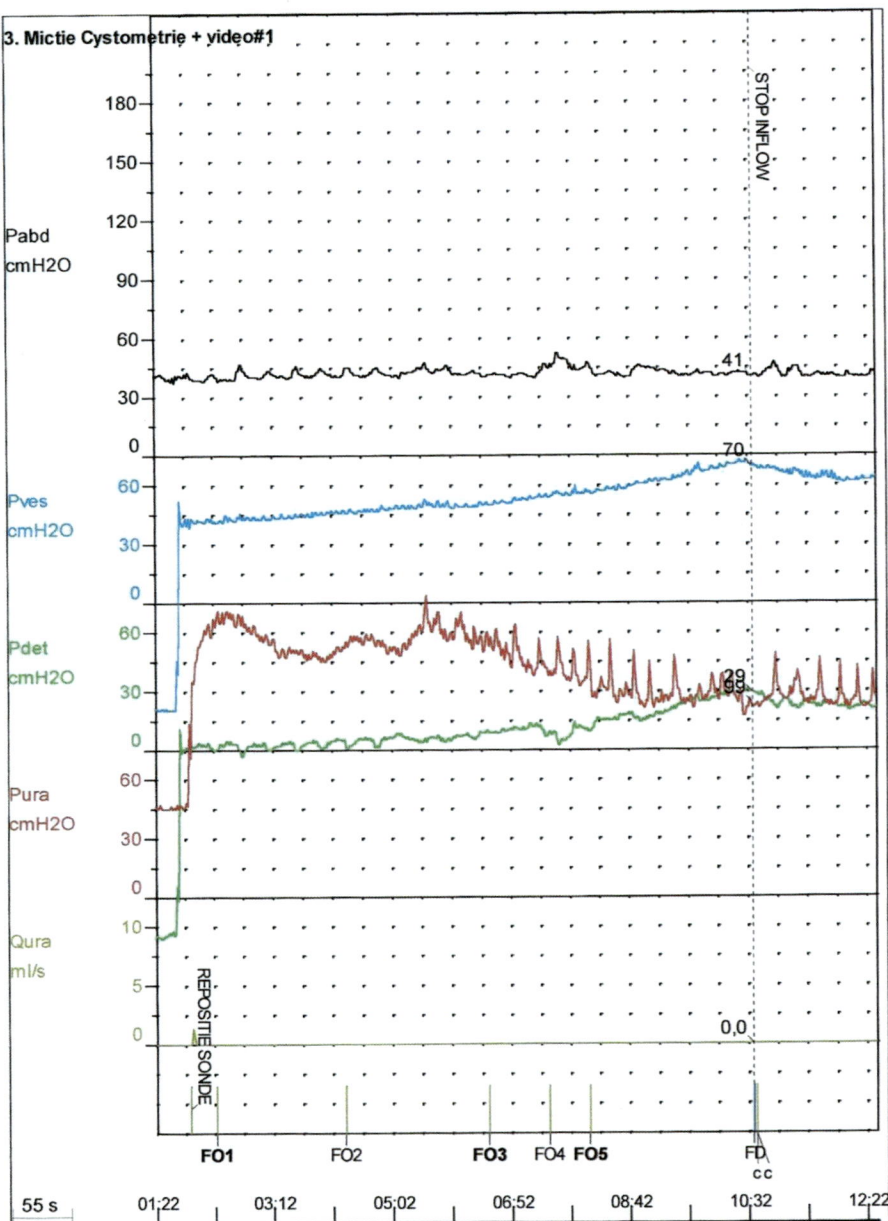

Fig. 17.14 Pdet at start = 0 cm H_2O. Filling rate 30 ml/min. Low pressure rises at the end of bladder filling in Pves and Pdet. After filling stopped Pdet decreases. Pdet pressure rise between start and end of filling, normal compliance (474/30=16). FD = first desire to void. ND = normal desire to void

Compliance during filling cystometry: 30 cm H$_2$O pressure rise from start to end filling: 474/30 = 16 ml/cm H$_2$O

Urethral Function: Very strong activity, high Pura

Maximum detrusor pressure: ___29_____ cm H$_2$O

Cystometric bladder capacity: ___474____ mL

Post void residual volume: _____no voiding

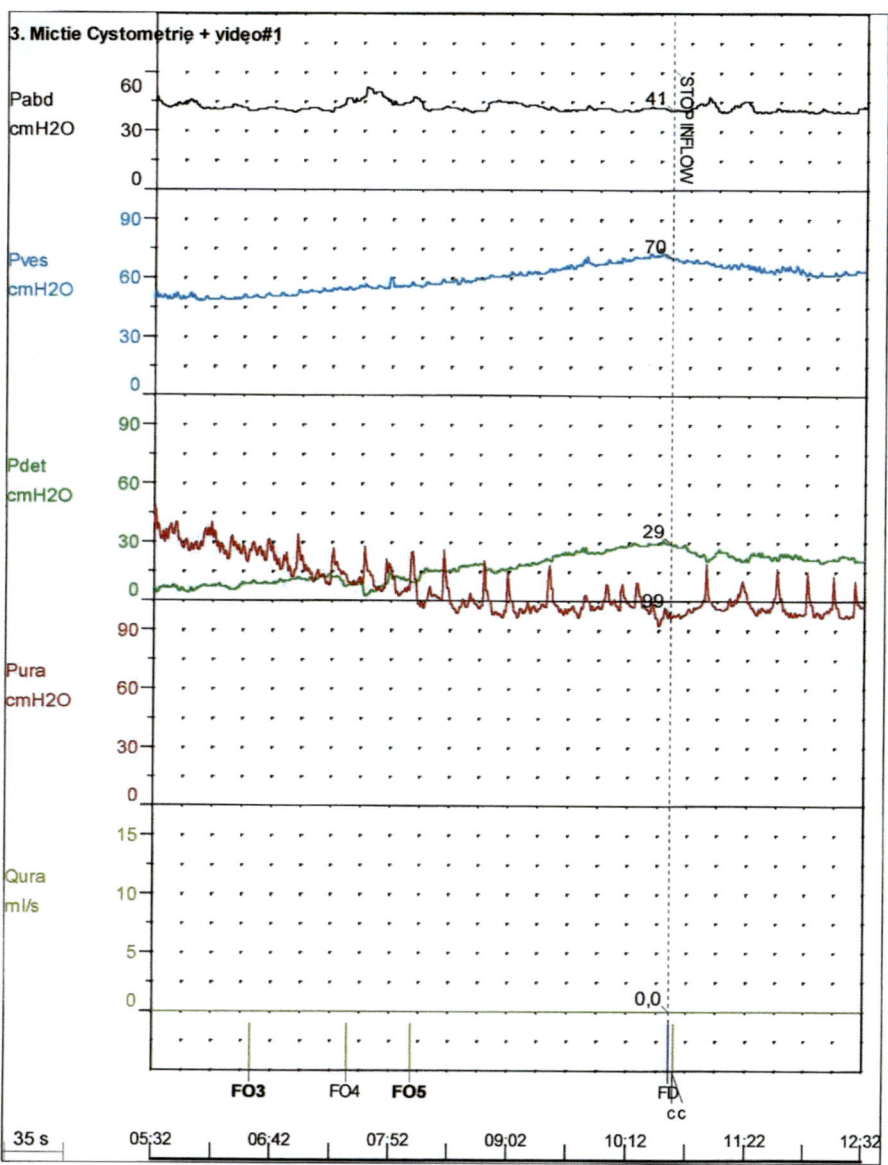

Fig. 17.15 Enlarged image of end of filling showing Pves and Pdet pressure rise. Pura high pressure with peaks. After stop filling gradually lowering of Pdet

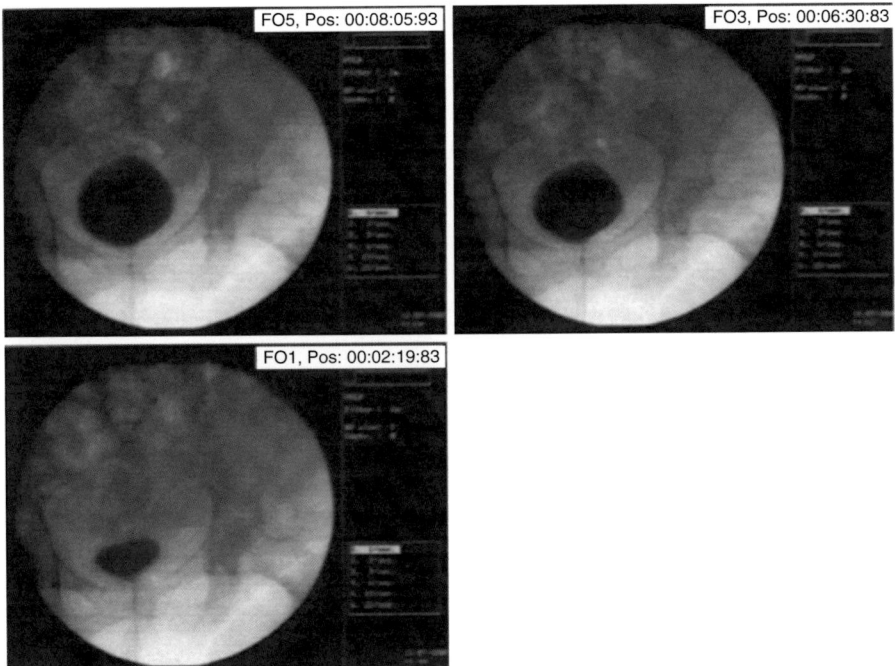

Fig. 17.16 Normal image of bladder, bladder neck closed. FO number = sequence of pictures taken. Not all pictures depicted here

17.6.4 Urinary Tract Imaging Basic Data Set (see Fig. 17.16)

Ultrasound of the urinary tract: Normal
X-ray of the urinary tract—Kidney Ureter Bladder: Normal at start of video-urodynamics (not depicted in Fig. 17.16)
Renography: Not done
Cystogram: Normal
Voiding cystogram: No voiding
Cystoscopy: Normal
Electrosensation bladder and urethra: No electrosensation in LUT

17.6.5 Management

Suprapubic catheter. If effect of botulinum toxin disappears, re-inject.

This case shows negative electrosensation but some filling sensation. This is possible because both sensations have different pathways.

17.7   Case 7

Figures 17.17 and 17.18

17.7.1 History

A 31 years old man, T2 paraplegia, AIS A.

    Road traffic accident 6 years ago. Fracture luxation C5–C6 with anterolisthesis: cervical fusion C5–C6. Central myelomalacy and syringo-hydromyelia. Posterior disco-osteophytic protrusion against cervical cord.

17.7.1.1   LUT Function Basic Data Set

Urinary tract impairment unrelated to spinal cord injury: No

Awareness of the need to empty the bladder: No

Bladder emptying: CISC and provoke micturition by tapping once per day with voiding of 200 ml

Average number of voluntary bladder emptyings per day during the last week: 3–5

Any involuntary urine leakage (incontinence) within the last three months: Yes, average daily 5–6 times

Collecting appliances for urinary incontinence: Diaper

Any drugs for the urinary tract within the last year: Antimuscarinics. Dosage doubled a month ago. Continence restored. Antibiotic for UTI. Antispastic drugs. Paracetamol

Surgical procedures on the urinary tract: No

Any change in urinary symptoms within the last year: Yes, incontinence worsened. Recurrent UTI.

Other: Laxative 3/week. Reflex erection. Increased spasticity lower limbs. No autonomic dysreflexia.

17.7.2 Clinical Examination

Sensation of touch perineum: absent. Cremaster reflex: positive both sides. Anal reflex: positive, bulbocavernosus reflex: positive. Voluntary contraction pelvic floor muscles: not possible.

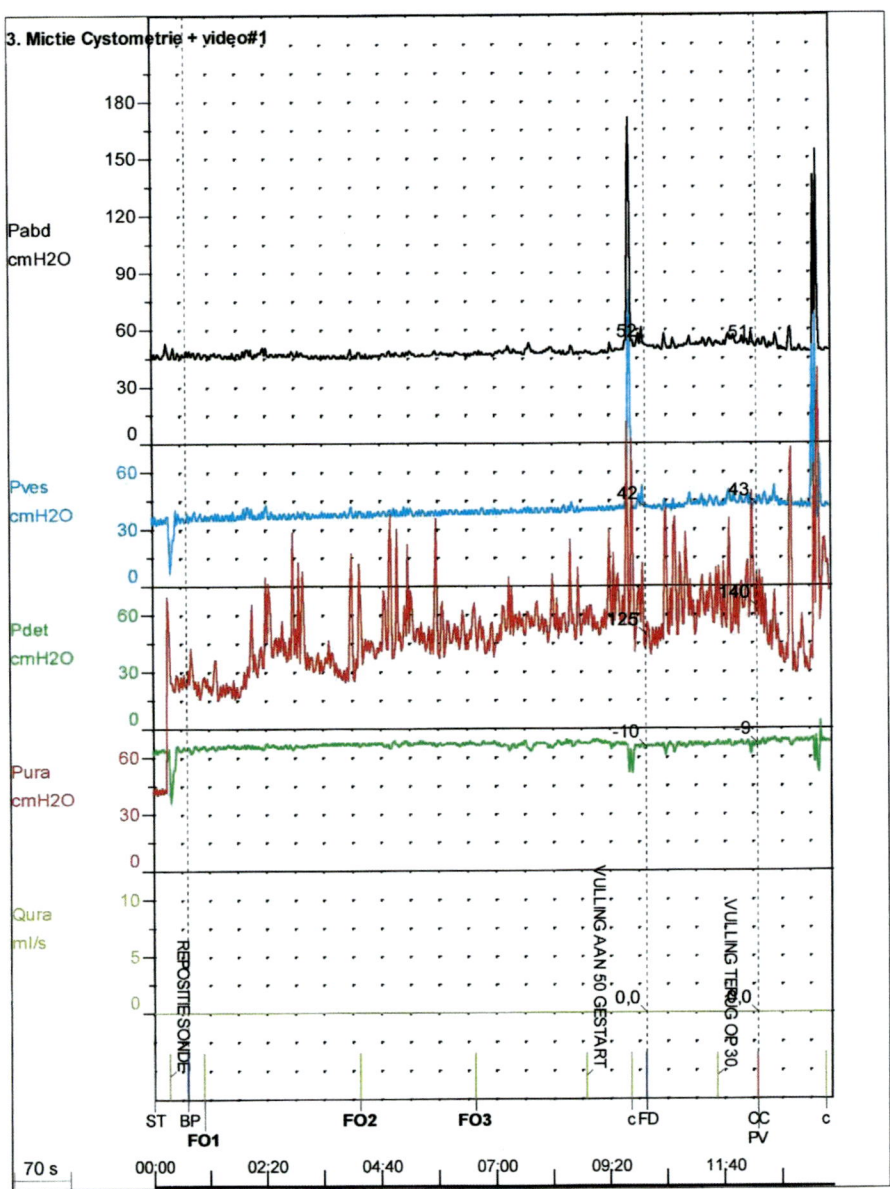

Fig. 17.17 Filling rate 30 ml/min. Pdet zeroing not correctly done as negative Pdet tracing shown. Slow pressure rise in Pves and Pabd. Pdet only little rise. Pura with high pressure and peaks. Increased Pura with cough and suprapubic tapping

17.7.3 Urodynamic Basic Data Set (see Fig. 17.17)

Bladder sensation during filling cystometry: Reduced. FDV at 325 ml
Detrusor function: Normal filling, no contraction.
Compliance during filling cystometry: Pdet rise of 4 cm H_2O, filling 421 ml = 105 ml/cm H_2O

Urethral function during voiding: No voiding
Maximum detrusor pressure: Difficult to calculate as zero Pdet is −14 cm H_2O
Cystometric bladder capacity: 421 mL
Post void residual volume: No voiding

17.7.4 Urinary Tract Imaging Basic Data Set (see Fig. 17.18)

Ultrasound of the urinary tract: Normal
X-ray of the urinary tract—Kidney Ureter Bladder: Normal at start of video-urodynamics
Renography: Not done
Cystogram: Normal
Voiding cystogram: No voiding, no leakage.

17.7.5 Other Diagnostic Tests

Cystoscopy: Strong spasticity of sphincter. Bladder wall trabeculation
Electrosensation: Present in LUT with higher threshold

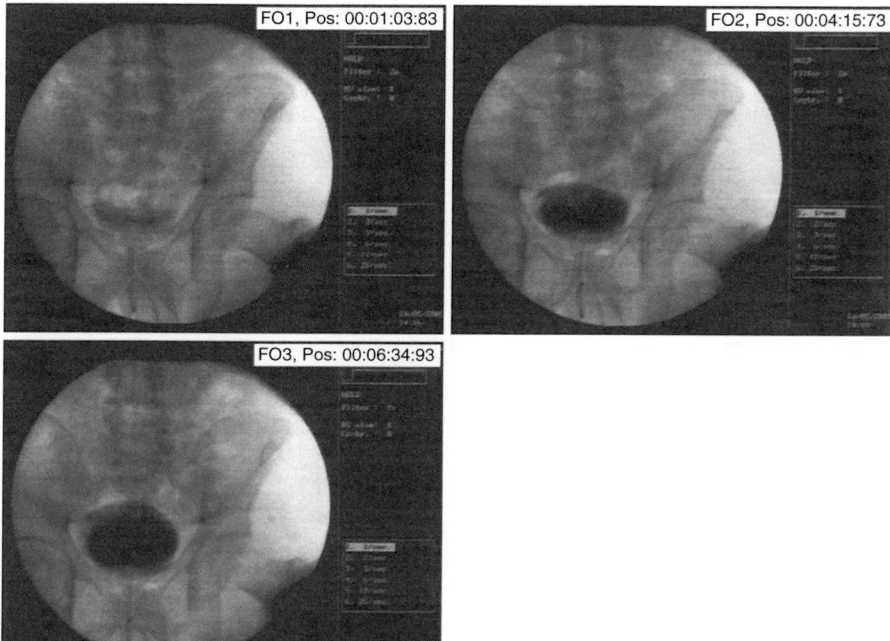

Fig. 17.18 Normal cystogram. FO number gives sequence of pictures taken. Not all depicted here

17.8   Case 8

Figure 17.19

17.8.1 History

A 28 years old man, T4 paraplegia, AIS A for 13 years

17.8.1.1   LUT Function Basic Data Set
Urinary tract impairment unrelated to spinal cord lesion: No
Awareness of the need to empty the bladder: No
Bladder emptying: Indwelling catheterization—transurethral
Any involuntary urine leakage within the last three months: No
Any drugs for the urinary tract within the last year: Anti-muscarinic, Oxybutynin
7.5 mg 3 times/day
Any change in urinary symptoms within the last year: No

17.8.2 Clinical Examination

Loss perianal and deep anal sense, positive BCR, tight sphincter tone, no voluntary
anal contraction (VAC).

17.8.3 Urodynamic Basic Data Set (see Fig. 17.19)

Bladder sensation during filling cystometry: No
Detrusor function: No involuntary detrusor contraction
Compliance during filling cystometry: Low (160/24, about 6 ml/cm H_2O)
Maximum detrusor pressure: 24 cm H_2O
Cystometric bladder capacity: 160 ml

Remark Infusion ends due to autonomic dysreflexia (AD) with BP rise to 160/96.
Small cystometric capacity is most likely due to prolonged indwelling catheterization. Antimuscarinic may help maintain or increase bladder capacity. In this case the
dosage may have to be increased.

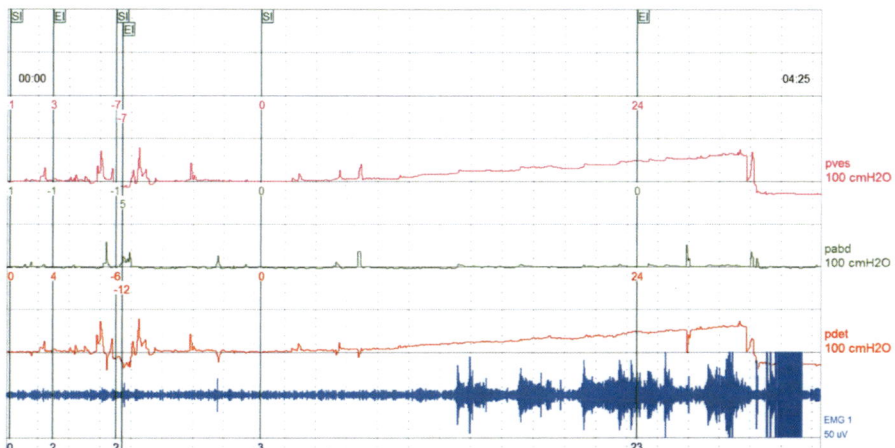

Fig. 17.19 Urodynamic tracings showing pressure rise of Pves but not of Pabd resulting in pressure rise only in Pdet without involuntary detrusor contraction indicating a low bladder compliance and a small cystometric capacity

17.9 Case 9

Figures 17.20 and 17.21

17.9.1 History

A 35 years old man, spastic T11 paraplegia, AIS B for 4 years

17.9.1.1 LUT Function Basic Data Set
Urinary tract impairment unrelated to spinal cord lesion: No
Awareness of the need to empty the bladder: No
Bladder emptying: CISC 6 times/d
Any involuntary urine leakage within the last three months: Yes, weekly
Any drugs for the urinary tract within the last year: No
Any change in urinary symptoms within the last year: No

17.9.2 Clinical Examination

Positive deep anal sense, BCR and anal reflex, normal sphincter tone, no voluntary anal contraction (VAC)

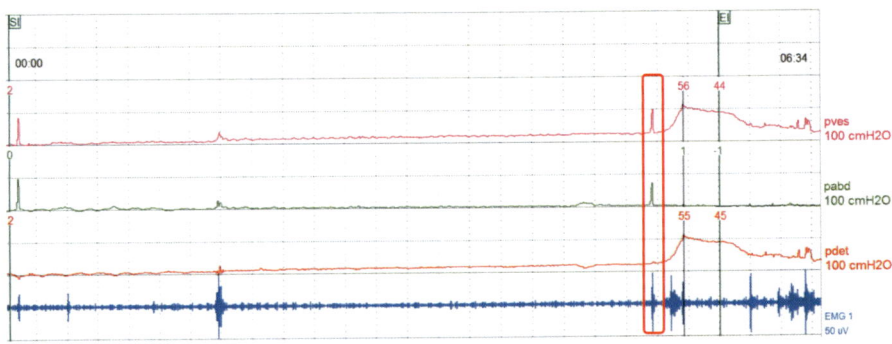

Fig. 17.20 A UDT shows terminal NDO starting at volume of 160 ml and Pdet of 10 cm H_2O with max Pdet of 55 cm H_2O

17.9.3 Urodynamic Basic Data Set (see Fig. 17.20)

Bladder sensation during filling cystometry: Unknown
Detrusor function: Terminal involuntary detrusor contraction
Compliance during filling cystometry: Normal (160/10 = 16 cm H_2O)
Maximum detrusor pressure: 55 cm H_2O
Cystometric bladder capacity: 210 ml

Remarks Coughing provokes detrusor contraction and also sphincter contraction (in red rectangular).

17.9.4 Management

Prescribe antimuscarinic, Trospium chloride 40 mg/d.

Request a repeated UDT a month later to evaluate the efficacy of antimuscarinic medication (see Fig. 17.21).

17.9.5 Follow-up

17.9.5.1 LUT Function Basic Data Set
Urinary tract impairment unrelated to spinal cord lesion: No
Awareness of the need to empty the bladder: No
Bladder emptying: CISC 6 times/d
Any involuntary urine leakage within the last three months: Yes, monthly but not weekly
Any drugs for the urinary tract within the last year: Antimuscarinic, Trospium chloride 40 mg/d for a month
Any change in urinary symptoms within the last year: Yes, less incontinence

17.9.5.2 Urine Strip
Sp.Gr. 1.005, pH 6.0, WBC 250, nitrite 2+, glucose –ve, blood –ve

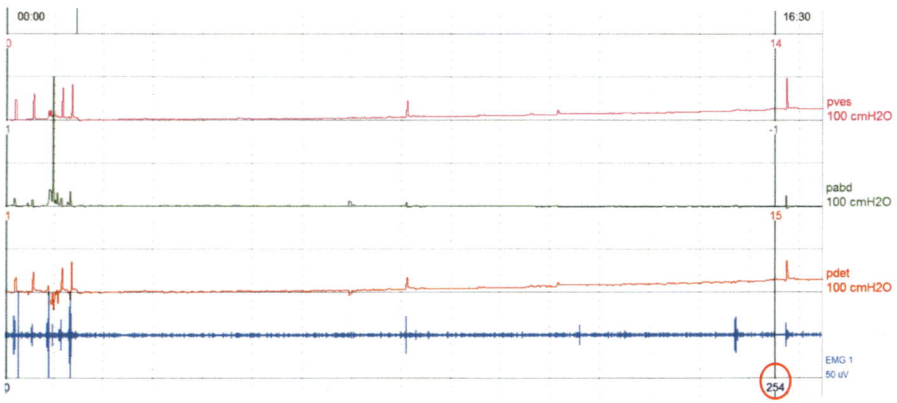

Fig. 17.21 A repeated UDT a month after taking antimuscarinic shows no involuntary detrusor contraction during filling cystometry, normal bladder sensations, max cystometric capacity of 450 ml with low Pdet reflecting normal compliance; no AD

17.9.5.3   Urodynamic Basic Data Set (see Fig. 17.21)

Bladder sensation during filling cystometry: Normal - first fillingat volume of 270 ml, first desire to void (FD) 360 ml, and strong desire to void (SF) 450 ml
Detrusor function: No involuntary detrusor contraction
Compliance during filling cystometry: Normal (450/15 = 30 ml/cm H_2O)
Maximum detrusor pressure: 15 cm H_2O
Cystometric bladder capacity: 450 ml

Remarks The infusion volume indicated in the tracing (in red circle) is less than the catheterised volume after the UDT ends. This might be due to poor calibration of the infusion pump and diuresis during UDT

17.9.5.4   Management

Continue antimuscarinic as the UDT shows no NDO with increase in cystometric capacity and bladder compliance.

Remarks Consider antibiotic prescription as urine strip shows evidence of UTI.

17.10 Case 10

Figures 17.22 and 17.23

17.10.1 History

A 28 years old man, SCI with spastic C5 tetraplegia, AIS C, onset Dec 2015
   Bladder over-distension (800 ml) during acute phase and failure to void

17.10.1.1 LUT Function Basic Data Set

Urinary tract impairment unrelated to spinal cord lesion: No
Awareness of the need to empty the bladder: Not known
Bladder emptying: Intermittent catheterization 5-6 times/d by nurse
Any involuntary urine leakage within the last three months: No
Any drugs for the urinary tract within the last year: Antibiotic for UTI
Any change in urinary symptoms within the last year: Yes, bladder over--distension and failure to void

17.10.2 Clinical Examination

Positive perianal sense, BCR, anal reflex, tight sphincter tone, and VAC

17.10.3 Urodynamic Basic Data Set (see Fig. 17.22)

Bladder sensation during filling cystometry: Normal, first desire to void (FD) at volume of 330 ml, strong desire to void (SD) at volume of 510 ml
Detrusor function: No involuntary detrusor contraction during filling and acontractile detrusor during voiding
Compliance during filling cystometry: Normal ($510/6 = 85$ ml/cm H_2O)
Maximum detrusor pressure: 6 cm H_2O
Cystometric bladder capacity: 510 ml
Urethral functions during voiding: Non-relaxing sphincter?

Remark Red arrow indicates end of infusion/filling phase. Waves of Pdet (in red rectangular) are artifacts, not involuntary contractions, but due to bowel movements. Tappings cause spikes in Pabd and Pves, and also increase spincter EMG. It is noted that the spikes of Pabd are higher than of Pves and this might be caused by sphincter contractions (in green rectangular) acting on rectal balloon placing not far enough from the anal sphincter. Straining increases both Pabd and Pves (in purple rectangular) but no voiding, perhaps due to not enough Pves with non-relaxing urethral sphincter obstruction.

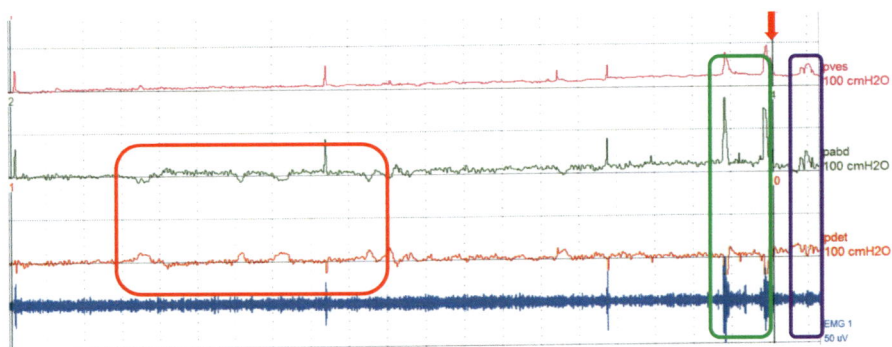

Fig. 17.22 The first UDT shows neither involuntary nor provoked detrusor contraction during filling phase and acontractile detrusor in voiding phase

17.10.4   Follow-up

After discharge, he could not void and decided to have indwelling catheterization.

Five months later, his motor function improves to AIS-D. A second UDT is requested.

17.10.4.1   LUT Function Basic Data Set

Urinary tract impairment unrelated to spinal cord lesion: No
Awareness of the need to empty the bladder: Not applicable
Bladder emptying: Indwelling transurethral catheterization with Foley catheter 14F, changed every 2 weeks
Any involuntary urine leakage within the last three months: No
Any drugs for the urinary tract within the last year: Antibiotic for UTI

17.10.4.2   Urine Strip

pH 7.0, Sp gr 1.005, WBC 25, negative nitrite

17.10.4.3   Urodynamic Basic Data Set (see Fig. 17.23)

Bladder sensation during filling cystometry: Increased, FD at volume of 250 ml, SD at volume of 300 ml
Detrusor function: No involuntary detrusor contraction during filling
Compliance during filling cystometry: Normal
Urethral functions during voiding: Initial DSD
Maximum detrusor pressure during voiding: 30 cm H_2O (underactive detrusor)
Cystometric bladder capacity: 300 ml

Remark Spikes in Pves and Pabd and increased EMG activity (in red rectangular) in voiding phase are due to straining. Spikes seen in Pabd but not in Pves (in purple rectangular) is due to removal of the urethral catheter.

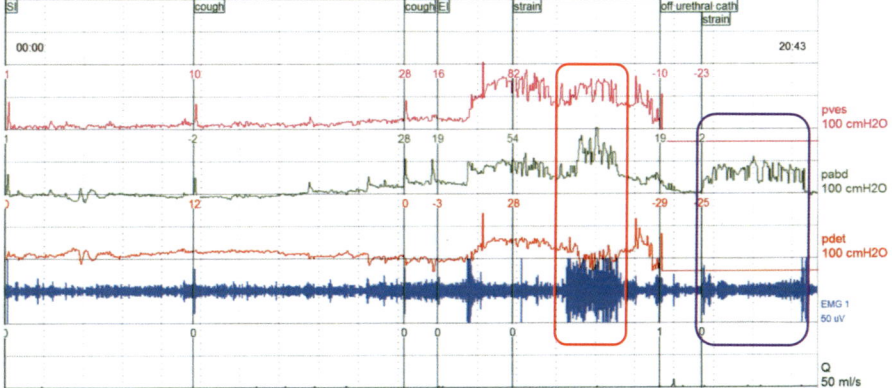

Fig. 17.23 Six months after onset, the UDT shows underactive detrusor with initial DSD and no voiding; when the urethral catheter is removed, voiding occurs but minimal

17.10.4.4 Management

Try straining and follow by CISC 4 times/day to empty the bladder.

17.11 Case 11

Figures 17.24 and 17.25

17.11.1 History

A 31 years old woman, T6 paraplegia, AIS B

17.11.1.1 LUT Function Basic Data Set

Urinary tract impairment unrelated to spinal cord lesion: No
Awareness of the need to empty the bladder: Yes
Bladder emptying: Voluntary void followed by CISC 6 times/d
Any involuntary urine leakage within the last three months: Yes
Any drugs for the urinary tract within the last year: No

17.11.2 Urodynamic Basic Data Set (see Fig. 17.24)

Bladder sensation during filling cystometry: Unknown
Detrusor function: Terminal involuntary detrusor contraction, max Pdet 70 cm H$_2$O with leakage

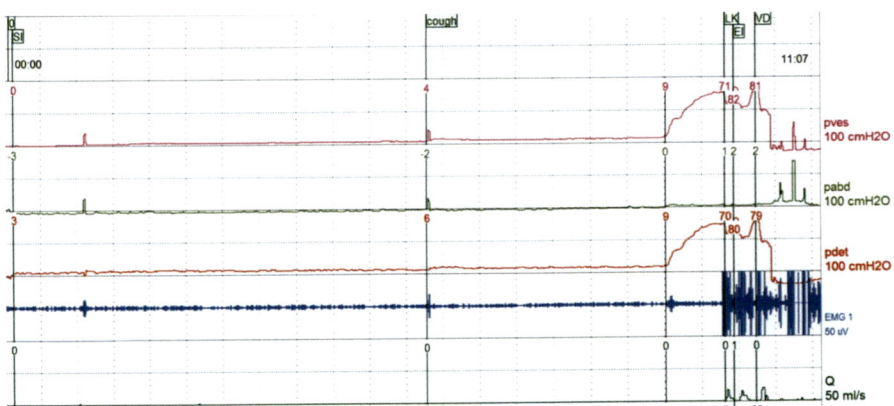

Fig. 17.24 The first UDT shows terminal detrusor overactivity (NDO) with leakage, small cystometric capacity, normal bladder compliance and intermittent voiding with low flow rate

Compliance during filling cystometry: Normal, 22 ml/cm H_2O
Urethral functions during voiding: DSD
Maximum detrusor pressure during voiding: 80 cm H_2O
Cystometric bladder capacity: 250 ml
Post-void residual volume: 150 ml

17.11.3 Management

Prescribe Tropium chloride 60 mg/d to reduce NDO and urinary incontinence.
   Continue CISC 6 times/d to completely empty the bladder.
   Repeat UDT to check drug efficacy.

17.11.4 Follow-up

Urinary incontinence persists but less.

17.11.4.1 LUT Function Basic Data Set
Urinary tract impairment unrelated to spinal cord lesion: No
Awareness of the need to empty the bladder: Yes
Bladder emptying: Voluntary voiding followed by CISC 6 times/d, PVR about 100 ml
Any involuntary urine leakage within the last three months: Yes but less than before
Any drugs for the urinary tract within the last year: Trospium chloride 60 mg/d to control NDO

17.11.4.2 Urine Strip
pH 5.0, Sp gr 1.010, nitrite –ve, WBC 25, glucose –ve, blood –ve

17.11.4.3 Urodynamic Basic Data Set (see Fig. 17.25)
Bladder sensation during filling cystometry: Increased, FD at 140 ml and SD at 170 ml
Detrusor function: Terminal and sustained involuntary detrusor contraction starting at volume of 180 ml
Compliance during filling cystometry: Normal (180/13 = 14 ml/cm H_2O)
Urethral functions during voiding: DSD
Maximum detrusor pressure during voiding: 57 cm H_2O with voided volume of 60 ml
Cystometric bladder capacity: 290 ml
Post-void residual volume: 230 ml

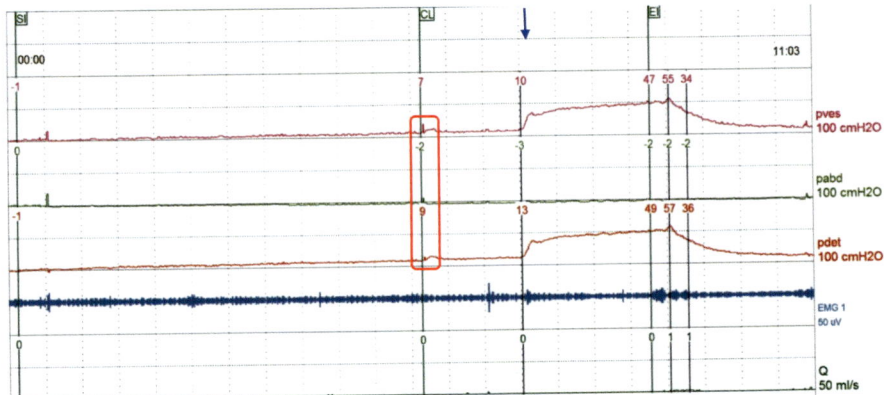

Fig. 17.25   A repeated UDT, three months later, shows sustained involuntary detrusor contraction starting at volume of 180 ml of strong desire to void (*blue arrow*)

Remark   Compared with the previous UDT, the NDO starts later with lower pressure. A low amplitude wave shown in Pves and Pdet after coughing indicates provoked detrusor contraction (in read rectangular), an evidence of NDO. Voiding is incomplete due to DSD and underactive detrusor. According to the ICS standards, detrusor underactivity is defined as a contraction of reduced strength and/or duration, resulting in prolonged bladder emptying and/or a failure to achieve complete bladder emptying within a normal time span.

17.11.4.4   Further Management
Increase the dosage of anti-muscarinic to Trospium chloride 80 mg/d to control urinary incontinence and detrusor contraction in order to prevent upper tract damage.

Continue CISC 6 times/d as voluntary voiding is inadequate.

17.12   Case 12

Figure 17.26

17.12.1   History

A 34 years old woman, transverse myeltitis with spastic C4 tetraplegia, AIS C for 16 years
     Sign of AD, rash at face, when bladder is full

17.12.1.1   LUT Function Basic Data Set

Urinary tract impairment unrelated to spinal cord lesion: No
Awareness of the need to empty the bladder: Yes, sometimes when having a strong desire to void
Bladder emptying: CIC by mother 4 times/d
Any involuntary urine leakage within the last three months: Yes
Any drugs for the urinary tract within the last year: Trospium chloride 80 mg/d to control NDO

17.12.2   Urodynamic Basic Data Set (see Fig. 17.26)

Bladder sensation during filling cystometry: Normal, FD at volume of 370 ml and SD at volume of 400 ml
Detrusor function: Terminal involuntary detrusor contraction (NDO)
Compliance during filling cystometry: Normal
Maximum detrusor pressure: 24 cm H_2O
Cystometric bladder capacity: 400 ml
Urethral functions during voiding: Not applicable due to no voiding phase

Remarks   Infusion is stopped due to increased BP indicating AD. There are no regularly coughs to check the responses of pressure transducers. The infused volume indicated when end of infusion (in green circle) is less than the catheterised volume at the end of the UDT. This might be due to diuresis and/or error of the infusion rate. Therefore it is recommended that pump calibration is performed regularly.

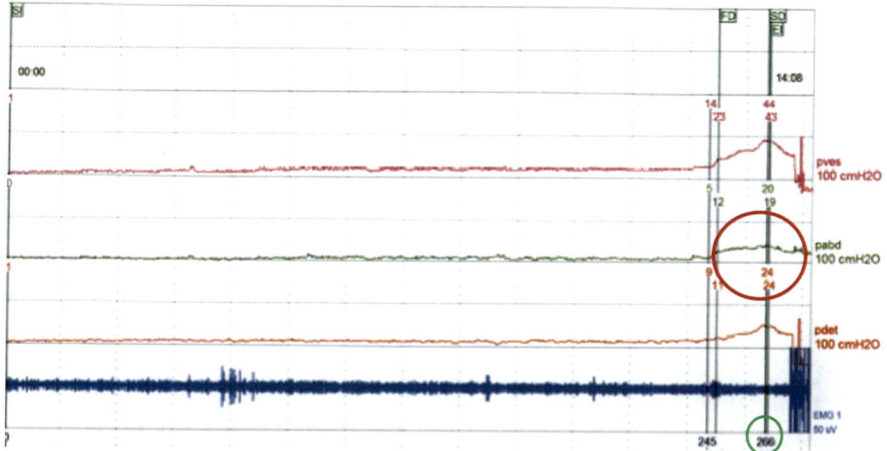

Fig. 17.26 This filling cystometry shows normal capacity, bladder compliance and terminal DO simultaneously with increased Pabd (in *red circle*) due to abdominal muscle spasm

17.13 Case 13

Figure 17.27

17.13.1 History

A 32 years old man, Guillain Barre syndrome with flaccid C4 tetraplegia, AIS D

17.13.1.1 LUT Function Basic Data Set
Urinary tract impairment unrelated to spinal cord lesion: No
Awareness of the need to empty the bladder: Yes
Bladder emptying: Voluntary void 200–300 ml per void, 4–5 times/d
Any involuntary urine leakage within the last three months: No but post-void dribbling
Any drugs for the urinary tract within the last year: No

17.13.2 Uroflowmetry

(Before UDT): Qmax/Vvoid/Vres = 40/550/90

17.13.3 Urodynamic Basic Data Set (see Fig. 17.27)

Bladder sensation during filling cystometry: Normal, FD at 300 ml and SD at 500 ml
Detrusor function: Normal, no involuntary contraction
Compliance during filling cystometry: Normal
Urethral functions during voiding: Non-relaxing sphincter
Maximum detrusor pressure during voiding: 13 cm H_2O
Cystometric bladder capacity: 500 ml

Remarks This patient cannot void when the filling catheter is in but after catheter removal, he voids 300 ml with mild straining. Due to high PVR (200 ml), urethral sphincter obstruction is suspected.

During voiding phase, removal of the filling catheter may be necessary to allow voiding possible when there is urethral sphincter obstruction.

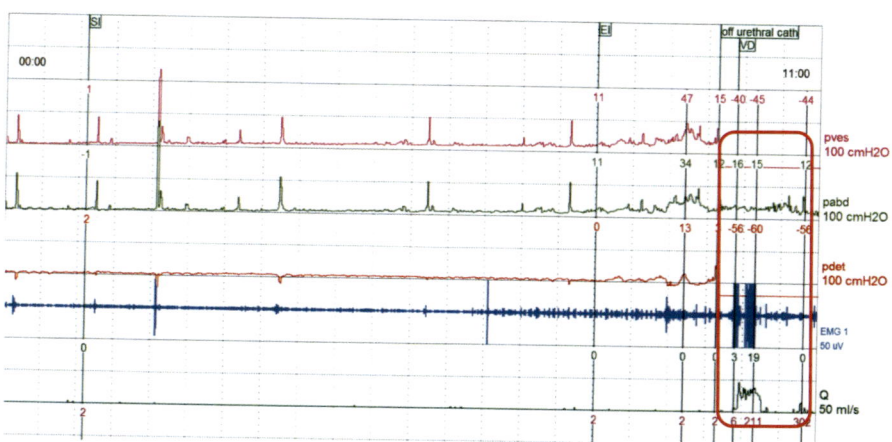

Fig. 17.27 Filling cystometry shows normal bladder compliance, detrusor function and urethral function; and voiding cystometry shows acontractile detrusor with non-relaxing sphincter, and no voiding; after removal of the urethral catheter (in red rectangular), voiding occurs with normal flow rate (19 ml/s) and mild straining (*low Pabd rise*)

17.14   Case 14

Figures 17.28 and 17.29

17.14.1   History

A 36 years old man, SCI with complete T12 paraplegia, AIS A

17.14.1.1   LUT Function Basic Data Set
Urinary tract impairment unrelated to spinal cord lesion: No
Awareness of the need to empty the bladder: No
Bladder emptying: CISC 4 times/d, volume per catheter 200–400 ml
Any involuntary urine leakage within the last three months: Yes, in between CISC
Any drugs for the urinary tract within the last year: No

17.14.2   Clinical Examination

Absent perianal and deep anal sensation, negative BCR and anal reflex, loose sphincter tone, no VAC

17.14.2.1   Urine Strip
pH 7.0, Sp gr. 1.015, WBC 25, nitrite 2+

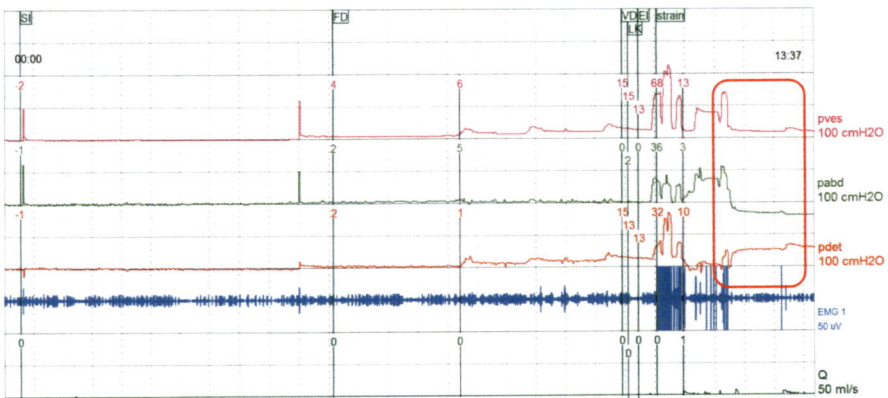

Fig. 17.28 Filling Cystometry shows NDO and voiding cystometry shows DSD with underactive detrusor and straining initiates intermittent voiding with low flow rate and prolonged voiding time

17.14.3   Urodynamic Basic Data Set (see Fig. 17.28)

Bladder sensation during filling cystometry: Increased, FD at 180 ml
Detrusor function: Phasic involuntary contraction starting at volume of 250, leakage occurs later
Compliance during filling cystometry: Normal
Urethral functions during voiding: DSD
Maximum detrusor pressure during voiding: 40 cm H_2O
Cystometric bladder capacity: 350 ml
Post-void residual volume: 280 ml

Remark   With a loose anal sphincter tone, straining can push the rectal catheter out, then the Pabd becomes negative and the Pdet is higher than it should be (in red rectangular). In this case, although neurological examination suggests sacral lesion but the UDT demonstrates NDO, most likely due to epiconal lesion.

17.14.4   Ultrasound of the Urinary Tract

Suspected bladder stone.

17.14.5   Management

Increase CISC frequency to prevent urinary incontinence. Refer to urologist for removal of bladder stone.

17.14.6   Follow-up

Cystolitholapraxy done 4 months later

17.14.6.1   Urine Strip

pH 5.0, Sp gr. 1.025, WBC 500, nitrite –ve, blood –ve

17.14.6.2   LUT Function Basic Data Set

Urinary tract impairment unrelated to spinal cord lesion: No
Awareness of the need to empty the bladder: Non-specific, abdominal discomfort
before catheterization sometime
Bladder emptying: CISC 4–5 times/d, volume per catheter – not measured
Any involuntary urine leakage within the last three months: Yes but less
Any drugs for the urinary tract within the last year: No

17.14.6.3   Clinical Examination

Absent perianal and deep anal sensation, weakly positive BCR and anal reflex, normal sphincter tone, no VAC

17.14.6.4   Urodynamic Basic Data Set (see Fig. 17.29)

Bladder sensation during filling cystometry: Normal, FD at volume of 250 ml,
SD at volume of 350 ml
Detrusor function: Phasic involuntary contraction starting at volume of 340 ml, no
leakage.
Compliance during filling cystometry: Normal
Urethral functions during voiding: Non-relaxing sphincter
Maximum detrusor pressure during voiding: 10 cm H_2O, no voiding
Cystometric bladder capacity: 390 ml
Remark   Compared with the previous UDT and neurological examination,
the first phasic involuntary contraction starting later at larger volume indicates
less active NDO which might be due to no stimulation/irritation from bladder
stone.

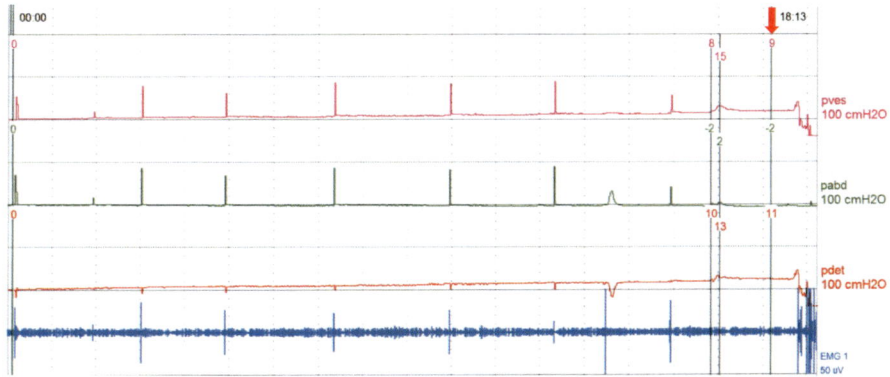

Fig. 17.29 This UDT demonstrates NDO starting at volume of 340 ml in filling cystometry and
acontractile detrusor in voiding cystometry. *Red arrow* indicates end of infusion. A *red arrow*
indicates end of infusion

17.15 Case 15

Figures 17.30 and 17.31

17.15.1 History

A 53 years old man, SCI with spastic T4 paraplegia, AIS A for 3 years

17.15.1.1   LUT Function Basic Data Set
Urinary tract impairment unrelated to spinal cord lesion: No
Awareness of the need to empty the bladder: No
Bladder emptying: Indwelling transurethral catheterization for 3 years, Foley catheter 16F
Any involuntary urine leakage within the last three months: When the catheter is blocked
Any drugs for the urinary tract within the last year: Trospium chloride 80 mg/d to relax bladder

17.15.2 Clinical Examination

No perianal or deep anal sensation, positive BCR and anal reflex, normal sphincter tone

17.15.2.1   Urine Strip
pH 5.0, Sp gr. 1.025, nitrite 2+, WBC 500

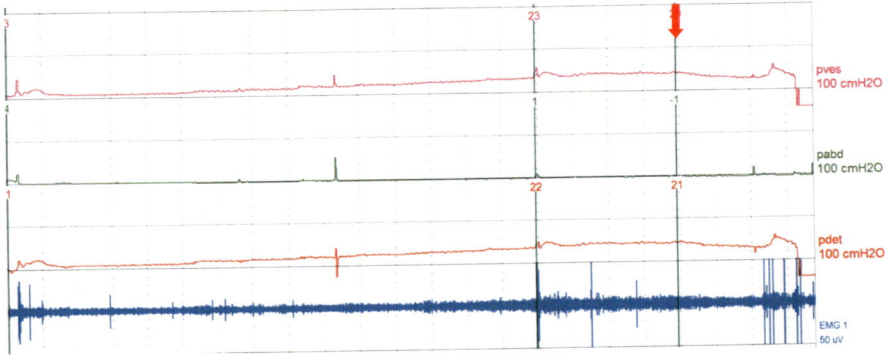

Fig. 17.30 Filling cystometry shows a low wave seen in Pves and Pdet after cough indicating provoked NDO. *Red arrow* indicates end of infusion

Fig. 17.31 Cystourethrogram performed by dripping of diluted contrast solution 280 ml into the urinary bladder via a Foley catheter and shows elongation of the urinary bladder with trabeculation and widening of the bladder neck, 1.9 cm in AP diameter. No vesicoureteral reflux is seen

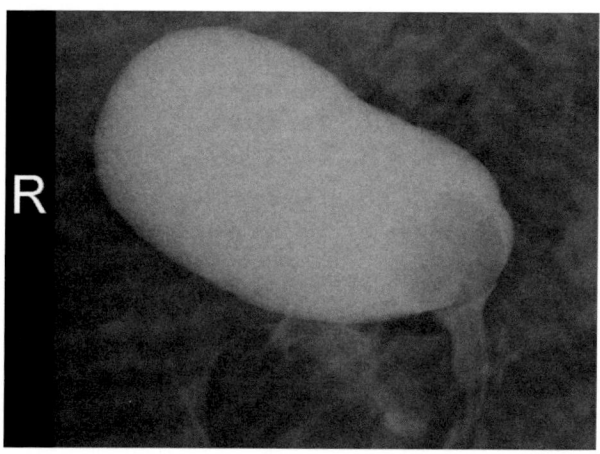

17.15.3   Urodynamic Basic Data Set (see Fig. 17.30)

Bladder sensation during filling cystometry: No
Detrusor function: Involuntary detrusor contraction after coughing
Compliance during filling cystometry: Normal
Cystometric capacity: 280 ml
Urethral functions during voiding: Not applicable
Maximum detrusor pressure during voiding: Not applicable

Remark   Infusion ends when blood pressure rises indicating AD (at red arrow).

17.15.4   Management

Continue trospium chloride 80 mg/d to maintain bladder capacity and compliance
    Continue indwelling catheterization according to leakage and patient's preference but avoid large catheter with large balloon.
    Request cystourethrogram to rule out bladder neck erosion and vesico-ureteral reflux (see Fig. 17.31).

17.15.4.1   Further Management
Continue same dosage of anti muscarinic.
    Advise the patient about other appropriate bladder management options better than transurethral indwelling catheterization to prevent further leakage around the catheter.
    Consult urologist.

17.16 Case 16

Figures 17.32 and 17.33

17.16.1 History

A 67 years old man, spastic C7 tetraplegia, AIS D. Three days before UDT, uroflowmetry showed nearly normal voiding (see Fig. 17.32)

17.16.1.1 LUT Function Basic Data Set
Urinary tract impairment unrelated to spinal cord lesion: No
Awareness of the need to empty the bladder: Yes
Bladder emptying: Voluntary voiding 150–400 ml/void
Any involuntary urine leakage within the last three months: No
Any drugs for the urinary tract within the last year: Doxazosin (2 mg) 1 tablet/d to relax bladder neck and Ofloxacin (200 mg) 1 × 2/d for treatment of UTI

17.16.2 Clinical Examination

Tight sphincter tone, weakly positive VAC, UEMS 34, LEMS 42, big toe flexor grade Rt 4/Lt 5

17.16.2.1 Urine Strip
pH 6.0, Sp. Gr. 1.010, nitrite –ve, WBC 250

17.16.3 Urodynamic Basic Data Set (see Figs. 17.32 and 17.33)

Bladder sensation during filling cystometry: Normal, FD at 460 ml and SD at 500 ml
Detrusor function: Terminal involuntary contraction with max Pdet of 34 cm H_2O
Compliance during filling cystometry: Normal
Urethral functions during voiding: Initial DSD
Maximum detrusor pressure during voiding: 34 cm H_2O
Cystometric bladder capacity: 500 ml
Post-void residual volume: 150 ml

Remark Slower flow rate and higher PVR during voiding cystometry than during uroflowmetry might be due to retained filling catheter when there is some degree of urethral sphincter obstraction.

17.16.4 Management

Continue the same dosage of Doxazosin.
  Void at the first desire to void to prevent bladder overdistension.
  Try double voiding to completely empty the bladder as much as possible.

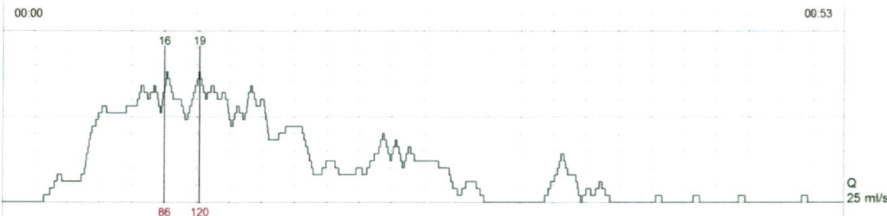

Fig. 17.32 Uroflowmety, three days before UDT, shows nearly normal voiding with Qmax/Vvoid/Vres = 19/260/10

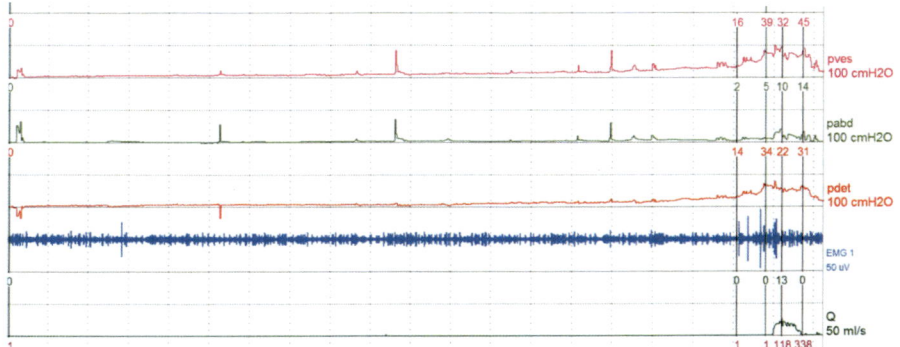

Fig. 17.33 Filling cystometry shows normal bladder compliance and cystometric capacity with terminal NDO; and voiding cystometry shows underactive detrusor with initial DSD and slow flow rate of 13 ml/sec

17.17   Case 17

Figures 17.34 and 17.35

17.17.1   History

A 57 years old man, old SCI with spastic T11 paraplegia, AIS A, for 5 years, prefers less CISC and accepts incontinence

17.17.1.1   LUT Function Basic Data Set

Urinary tract impairment unrelated to spinal cord lesion: No
Awareness of the need to empty the bladder: No
Bladder emptying: CISC 5 times/d, volume per catheter 100–200 ml
Any involuntary urine leakage within the last three months: Yes, about 1 L/d, need condom during the day
Any drugs for the urinary tract within the last year: Oxybutynin 15 mg/d to relax bladder, Doxazocin 2 mg/d

17.17.2   Urodynamic Basic Data Set (see Fig. 17.34)

Bladder sensation during filling cystometry: No
Detrusor function: Phasic involuntary contractions staring at volume of 100 ml, max Pdet 52 cm H$_2$O with leakage
Compliance during filling cystometry: Low (at cystometric capacity)
Urethral functions during voiding: Suspected DSD
Maximum detrusor pressure during voiding: Not applicable
Cystometric bladder capacity: 300 ml

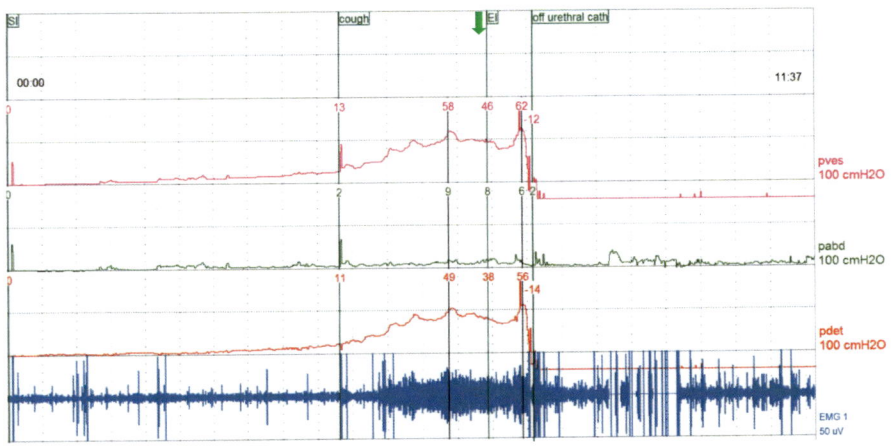

Fig. 17.34 This UDT demonstrates NDO with low bladder compliance

17.17.3   Follow-up

Due to dry mouth, he reduced the dosage of oxybutynin to 10 mg/d and did CISC 5 times/d and applied a condom to collect leakage as usual. A follow-up UDT was done a year later (see Fig. 17.35).

17.17.3.1   Urine Strip
pH 8.0, Sp Gr 1.000, nitrite –ve, WBC 25, blood –ve, sugar –ve

17.17.3.2   Urodynamic Basic Data Set (see Fig. 17.35)
Bladder sensation during filling cystometry: Absent
Detrusor function: Terminal involuntary contraction staring at volume of 150 ml, max Pdet 119 cm H_2O with leakage
Compliance during filling cystometry: Normal (150/5 = 30 ml/cm H_2O)
Urethral functions during voiding: Not applicable due to no voiding but suspected DSD
Maximum detrusor pressure during voiding: Not applicable
Cystometric bladder capacity: 150 ml

Remark   Very high Pdet might be due to less dosage of oxybutynin. To be noted, the specific gravity of the urine is 1.000 reflecting a lot of fluid intake before UDT and dieresis might occur during UDT. In addition, according to the ICS standards for calculation of the bladder compliance, in this case one should use the Pves, not the Pdet, immediate before the start of the detrusor contraction that causes significant leakage because the Pdet is lower than it should be due to rising of Pabd from bowel movement (in a red rectangular).

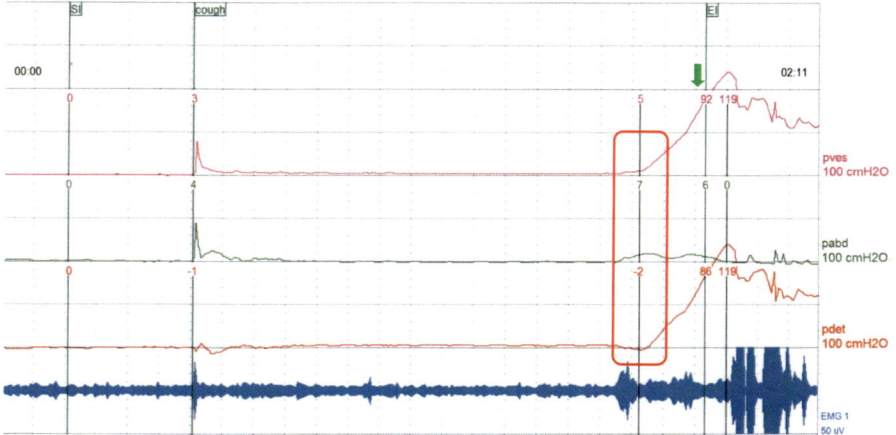

Fig. 17.35 This UDT done a year later shows strong terminal NDO with very high Pdet (over 100 cm H_2O) and leakage (a *green arrow*) and small cystometric capacity

17.17.4 Management

Discontinue doxazocin to reduce incontinence.

Increase the dosage of oxybutynin to 30 mg/d, if not tolerable, switch to trospium chloride 80 mg/d.

Increase CISC frequency according to volume of fluid intake.

17.18 Case 18

Figures 17.36 and 17.37

17.18.1 History

A 54 years old man, SCI with incomplete L2 paraplegia, AIS C, walks with forearm crutches for more than 20 years.

17.18.1.1 LUT Function Basic Data Set

Urinary tract impairment unrelated to spinal cord lesion: No
Awareness of the need to empty the bladder: Yes, non-specific with abdominal discomfort
Bladder emptying: CISC 4 times/d, volume per catheter 300–400 ml
Any involuntary urine leakage within the last three months: Yes, sometimes
Any drugs for the urinary tract within the last year: No

17.18.2 Clinical Examination

Diminished perianal sensation, positive deep anal sensation; positive BCR and anal reflex; positive VAC.

LEMS 24, big toe flexors—gr 0

17.18.2.1 Urine Strip

pH 6.0, Sp Gr 1.025, WBC 75, nitrite –ve

17.18.3 Urodynamic Basic Data Set (see Fig. 17.36)

Bladder sensation during filling cystometry: Yes
Detrusor function: No involuntary contractions but suspected provoked NDO?
Compliance during filling cystometry: Normal
Urethral functions during voiding: Not applicable
Maximum detrusor pressure during voiding: Not applicable
Cystometric bladder capacity: 400 ml

Remark   Provoked NDO (in a red rectangular) is suspected.

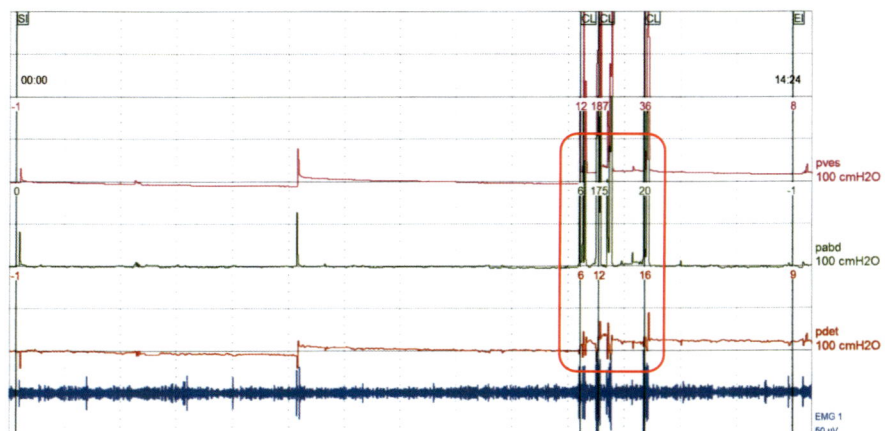

Fig. 17.36 This UDT demonstrates strong coughs with very high Pves and Pabd and increased sphincter EMG activity but no leakage

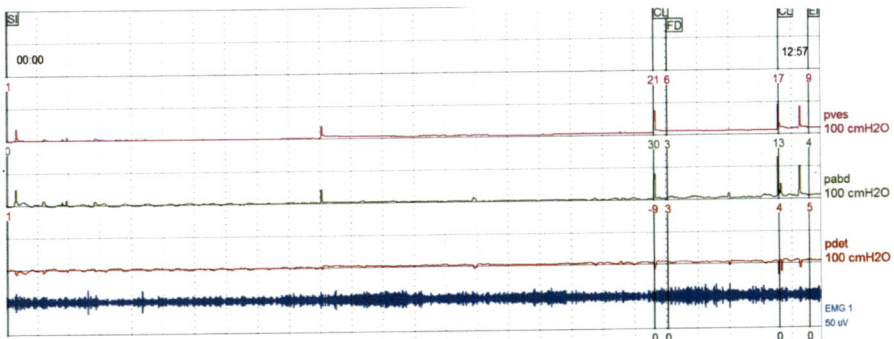

Fig. 17.37 This UDT shows normal filling cystometry

17.18.4 Follow-up

Two years later, he comes for check-up and reports no change in bladder management and no UTI.

17.18.4.1   Urine Strip
pH 6.0, Sp Gr 1.030, WBC 25, nitrite 1+

17.18.4.2   Urodynamic Basic Data Set (see Fig. 17.37)
Bladder sensation during filling cystometry: Normal, at volume of 250 ml and SD at 310 ml
Detrusor function: Normal
Compliance during filling cystometry: Normal
Urethral functions during voiding: Not applicable
Maximum detrusor pressure during voiding: Not applicable
Cystometric bladder capacity: 340 ml

17.18.5 Management

Continue CISC 4–5 times/d when having a strong desire to void
Prescribe a new silicone self catheter set and change it yearly, and change antiseptic solution daily to reduce risk of UTI

17.19 Case 19

Figures 17.38 and 17.39

17.19.1 History

A 35 years old man, SCI with complete spastic T11 paraplegia, AIS A, for 4 years

17.19.1.1 LUT Function Basic Data Set
Urinary tract impairment unrelated to spinal cord lesion: No
Awareness of the need to empty the bladder: No
Bladder emptying: Transurethral indwelling catheterization, change Foley catheter weekly by nurse
Any involuntary urine leakage within the last three months: No
Any drugs for the urinary tract within the last year: No

17.19.2 Clinical Examination

No deep anal sensation, negative BCR and anal reflex, LEMS 0, big toe flexor gr 0

17.19.2.1 Urine Strip
pH 7.0, Sp. Gr. 1.005, WBC 250, nitrite 2+

17.19.3 Urodynamic Basic Data Set (see Fig. 17.38)

Bladder sensation during filling cystometry: Increased, FD at volume of 47 ml
Detrusor function: Terminal involuntary contractions staring at small filling volume, Pdet 15 cm H_2O with leakage 30 ml
Compliance during filling cystometry: Low
Urethral functions during voiding: Not applicable
Maximum detrusor pressure during voiding: Not applicable
Cystometric bladder capacity: 90 ml (catheterised volume after UDT ends)

Remark Combining an early NDO with urine strip showing bacteriuria and pyuria, UTI should be suspected.

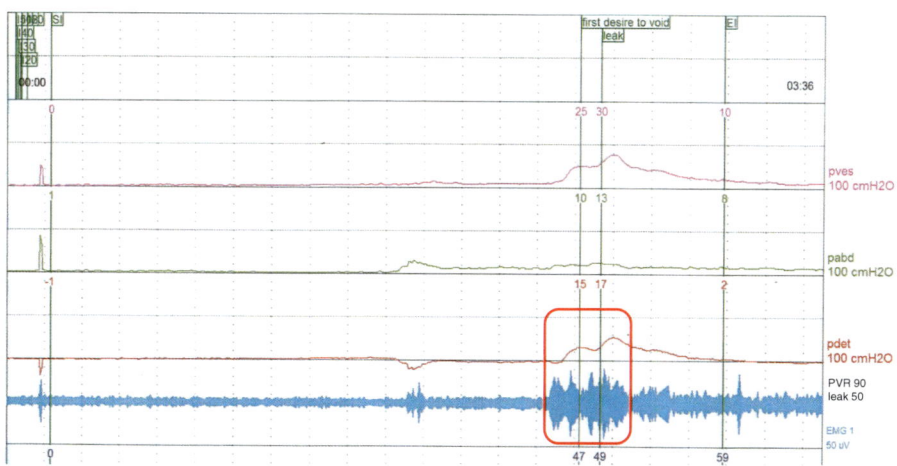

Fig. 17.38 This UDT demonstrates terminal NDO simultaneously with increased sphincter EMG activity (in a *red rectangular*)

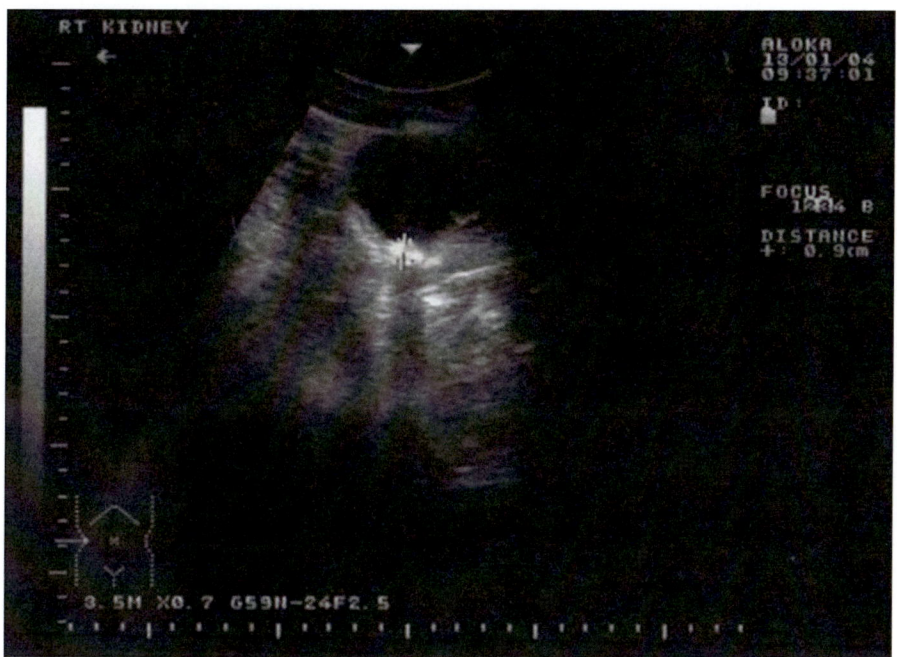

Fig. 17.39 Calcification with acoustic shadow indicates bladder stone

17.19.4   Ultrasound of the Urinary Tract (see Fig. 17.39)

No kidney stone, normal size of both kidneys, no hydronephrosis but bladder stone 0.9 × 3.3 cm is detected

17.19.5 Management

Start oxybutynin 15 mg/d to control NDO and increase bladder capacity.
Consult urologist for removal of the bladder stone.
Repeat UDT after bladder stone removal to evaluate the effect of oxybutynin.
Change to CISC if bladder capacity increases to 200–300 ml.

17.20 Case 20

Figure 17.40

17.20.1 History

A 53 years old woman, secondary progressive multiple sclerosis for 5 years
About three weeks after this 4th attack with spastic tetraplegia C5 and no voiding,
a UDT is requested.

17.20.1.1 LUT Function Basic Data Set
Urinary tract impairment unrelated to spinal cord lesion: No
Awareness of the need to empty the bladder: No
Bladder emptying: Transurethral indwelling catheterization, change Foley catheter weekly by nurse
Any involuntary urine leakage within the last three months: No
Any drugs for the urinary tract within the last year: No

17.20.2 Clinical Examination

No deep anal sensation, negative BCR and anal reflex, loose sphincter tone; UEMS 32, LEMS 0, no VAC

17.20.2.1 Urine Strip
pH 5.0, Sp. Gr. 1.010, WBC 75, nitrite –ve

17.20.3 Urodynamic Basic Data Set (see Fig. 17.40)

Bladder sensation during filling cystometry: Absent
Detrusor function: Phasic involuntary contractions, Pdet 38 cm H_2O with leakage 10 ml

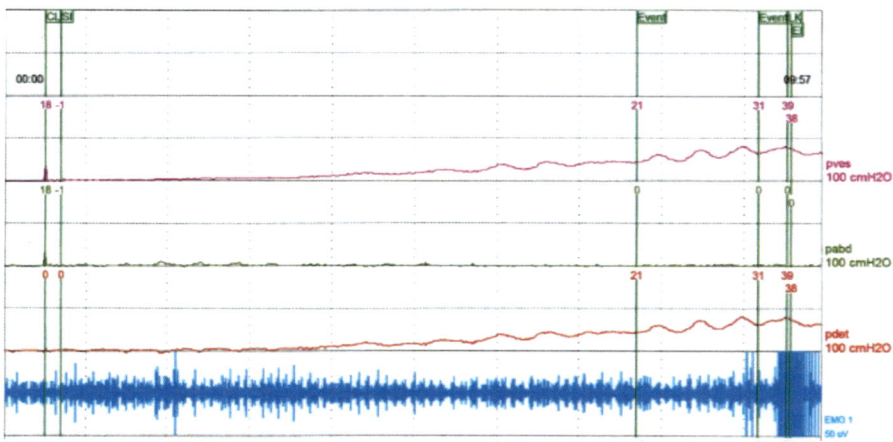

Fig. 17.40   This filling cystometry demonstrate NDO with minimal leakage at the end of the UDT

Compliance during filling cystometry: Low (250/30 = 8 ml/cm H_2O)
Urethral functions during voiding: Not applicable
Maximum detrusor pressure during voiding: Not applicable
Cystometric bladder capacity: 250 ml (catheterised volume after UDT ends)

Remark   Failure to void is suspected to be due to DSD.

17.20.4   Management

Discontinue Foley catheter and start intermittent catheterization 4–6 times/d according to bladder diary.

Prescribe low dose of oxybutynin (7.5 mg/d) to control NDO, and prevent leakage after the Foley catherter is removed.

Data Sets

The purpose of the Lower Urinary Tract Function, Urodynamic and Urologic Imaging Basic Data Set is to standardize the collection and reporting of a minimal amount of information on the lower urinary tract in daily practice. Their use makes it possible to evaluate and compare results from various studies.

The urologic datasets are some of a long list of data sets on most aspects of SCI management. They can be downloaded for free from www.iscos.org.uk

Referencing should be done as

International LUT function basic SCI data set. Spinal Cord 2008;46:325–330.

International urodynamic basic SCI data set. Spinal Cord 2008;46:513–516

International urinary tract imaging basic SCI data set. Spinal Cord 2009;47:379–383.

© Springer International Publishing AG 2017
J.J. Wyndaele, A. Kovindha, *Urodynamic Testing After Spinal Cord Injury*,
DOI 10.1007/978-3-319-54900-2_18

18.1   Lower Urinary Tract Function Basic Data Set

Date of data collection: YYYYMMDD

Urinary tract impairment unrelated to spinal cord injury:

- ☐   No
- ☐   Yes, specify_____
- ☐   Unknown

Awareness of the need to empty the bladder:

- ☐   No
- ☐   Yes
- ☐   Not applicable
- ☐   Not known

Bladder emptying:

		Main	Supplement
☐	Normal voiding	☐	☐
☐	Bladder reflex triggering		
☐	Voluntary (tapping, scratching, anal stretch, etc.)	☐	☐
☐	Involuntary	☐	☐
☐	Bladder expression		
☐	Straining (abdominal straining, Valsalva's manoeuvre)	☐	☐
☐	External compression (Credé manoeuvre)	☐	☐
☐	Intermittent catheterization		
☐	Self-catheterization	☐	☐
☐	Catheterization by attendant	☐	☐
☐	Indwelling catheter		
☐	Transurethral	☐	☐
☐	Suprapubic	☐	☐
☐	Sacral anterior root stimulation	☐	☐
☐	Non-continent urinary diversion/ostomy	☐	☐
☐	Other method, specify_____	☐	☐
☐	Unknown		

Average number of voluntary bladder-emptyings per day during the last week__

Any involuntary urine leakage (incontinence) within the last three months:

☐ No

☐ Yes, average daily

☐ Yes, average weekly

☐ Yes, average monthly

☐ Not applicable   ☐ Unknown

Collecting appliances for urinary incontinence:

☐ No

☐ Yes, condom catheter

☐ Yes, diaper

☐ Yes, ostomy bag

☐ Yes, other, specify_____

☐ Unknown

Any drugs for the urinary tract within the last year:

☐ No

☐ Yes, bladder relaxant drugs (anticholinergics, tricyclic antidepressants, etc.)

☐ Yes, sphincter/bladder neck relaxant drugs (alpha adrenergic blockers, etc.)

☐ Yes, antibiotics/antiseptics:

　　☐ For treatment of urinary tract infection

　　☐ For prophylactic reasons

☐ Yes, other, specify_____

☐ Unknown

Surgical procedures on the urinary tract:

☐ No

☐ Yes, supra-pubic catheter insertion, date last performed YYYYMMDD

☐ Yes, bladder stone removal, date last performed YYYYMMDD

☐ Yes, upper urinary tract stone removal, date last performed YYYYMMDD

☐ Yes, bladder augmentation, date last performed YYYYMMDD

☐ Yes, sphincterotomy/urethral stent, date last performed YYYYMMDD

☐ Yes, botulinum toxin injection, date last performed YYYYMMDD

☐ Yes, artificial sphincter, date last performed YYYYMMDD

☐ Yes, ileovesicostomy urinary diversion, date last performed YYYYMMDD

☐ Yes, ileoureterostomy, date last performed YYYYMMDD

☐ Yes, continent vesicostomy, date last performed YYYYMMDD

☐ Yes, sacral anterior root stimulator, date performed YYYYMMDD

☐ Yes, other, specify_____ , date performed YYYYMMDD

☐ Unknown

Any change in urinary symptoms within the last year:

☐ No

☐ Yes

☐ Not applicable

☐ Unknown

18.2　Urodynamic Basic Data Set

Date performed: YYYYMMDD

☐ Unknown

Bladder sensation during filling cystometry:

☐ Normal

☐ Increased

☐ Reduced

☐ Absent

☐ Non-specific

☐ Unknown

Detrusor function

☐ Normal

☐ Neurogenic detrusor overactivity

☐ Acontractile detrusor

☐ Unknown

Compliance during filling cystometry:

Low (< 10 mL/cm H20)

☐ Yes

☐   No

☐   Unknown

Function during voiding:

☐   ☐ Normal   ☐ Detrusor sphincter dyssynergia   ☐ Not applicable ☐ Unknown

☐   **Detrusor leak point pressure**_____ cm H2O   ☐ Not applicable ☐ Unknown

☐   **Maximum detrusor pressure**_____ cm H2O   ☐ Not applicable   ☐ Unknown

☐   **Cystometric bladder capacity**_____ mL

☐   ☐ Not applicable ☐ Unknown

☐   **Post void residual volume**_____ mL

☐   ☐ Not applicable ☐ Unknown

18.3   Urinary Tract Imaging Basic Data Set

Intravenous pyelography / Urography or CT urogram, or Ultrasound of the urinary tract

Date performed: YYYYMMDD

Method used:

☐   Intravenous pyelography / Urography

☐   CT urography

☐   Ultrasound of the urinary tract

☐   Normal

☐   Stasis/dilatation in upper urinary tract: ☐ Right side   ☐ Left side

☐   Kidney stone: ☐ Right side   ☐ Left side

☐   Stone in ureter: ☐ Right side   ☐ Left side

☐   Bladder stone

☐   Other findings:_____

X-ray of the urinary tract - Kidney Ureter Bladder (KUB)

Date performed: YYYYMMDD

☐   Normal

Kidney stone: ☐ Right side   ☐ Left side

Stone in ureter: ☐ Right side   ☐ Left side

☐   Bladder stone

☐   Other findings:_____

Renography

Date performed: YYYYMMDD

Method used:

- – ☐   DMSA (Technetium-99m dimercaptosuccinic acid)

- – ☐   DTPA (Technetium-99m diethylenetriamine pentaacetic acid)

- – ☐   Mag 3 (Technetium-99m mercaptoacetyltriglycine)

☐ Normal

- Excretory function: Right side ___% 　Left side ___%

- Stasis/dilatation in upper urinary tract: ☐ Right side ☐ Left side

☐ Other findings:_

Clearance

Date performed: YYYYMMDD

_____mL/(min. x 1.73 m^2)

Cystogram

Date performed: YYYYMMDD

☐ Normal

☐ Bladder stone

☐ Vesicoureteric reflux: ☐ Right ☐ Left

☐ Bladder diverticulum

☐ Bladder neck at rest: ☐ Open   ☐ Closed

☐ Other findings:_____

Voiding cystogram / Micturition cystourogram (MCU) / Videourodynamic

Date performed: YYYYMMDD

☐   Normal

☐   Vesicoureteric reflux: ☐ Right ☐ Left

☐   Bladder neck during voiding: ☐ Normal   ☐ Closed (dyssynergia)

☐   Striated urethral sphincter during voiding: ☐ Normal   ☐ Closed (dyssynergia)

☐   Other findings:_____

References

1. Schuld C, Franz S, van Hedel HJ, et al. International standards for neurological classification of spinal cord injury: classification skills of clinicians versus computational algorithms. Spinal Cord. 2015;53:324–31.
2. Wyndaele JJ. The normal pattern of perception of bladder filling during cystometry studied in 38 young healthy volunteers. J Urol. 1998;160:479–81.
3. Rossier AB, Fam BA, Dibenedetto M, Sarkarati M. Urodynamics in spinal shock patients. J Urol. 1979;122:783–7.
4. Wyndaele M, De Winter BY, Pelckmans PA, et al. Exploring associations between lower urinary tract symptoms (LUTS) and gastrointestinal (GI) problems in women: a study in women with urological and GI problems vs a control population. BJU Int. 2015;115:958–67.
5. Costa P, Perrouin-Verbe B, Colvez A, et al. Quality of life in spinal cord injury patients with urinary difficulties. Development and validation of qualiveen. Eur Urol. 2001;39:107–13.
6. Wyndaele M, De Winter BY, Van Roosbroeck S, et al. Development and psychometric evaluation of a dutch questionnaire for the assessment of anorectal and lower urinary tract symptoms. Acta Gastroenterol Belg. 2011;74:295–303.
7. Wyndaele JJ, THi HV, Pham BC, et al. The use of one-channel water cystometry in patients with a spinal cord lesion: practicalities, clinical value and limitations for the diagnosis of neurogenic bladder dysfunction. Spinal Cord. 2009;47:526–30.
8. Geirsson G, Lindstrom S, Fall M. Pressure, volume and infusion speed criteria for the ice-water test. Br J Urol. 1994;73:498–503.
9. Wyndaele JJ, Kovindha A, Madersbacher H, et al. Neurologic urinary and faecal incontinence. In: Abrams P, Cardozo L, Khoury S, Wein A, editors. Incontinence. 4th ed. Paris: Health Publication Ltd; 2009. p. 793–960.
10. Van Meel T, De Wachter S, Wyndaele JJ. Repeated ice water tests and electrical perception threshold determination to detect a neurologic cause of detrusor overactivity. Urology. 2007;70:772–6.
11. Sidi AA, Dijkstra DP, Peng W. Bethanechol supersensitivity test, rhabdosphincter electromyography and bulbocavernosus reflex latency in the diagnosis of neuropathic detrusor areflexia. J Urol. 1988;140:335–7.
12. Wyndaele JJ. Investigation of the afferent nerves of the lower urinary tract in patients with 'complete' and 'incomplete' spinal cord injury. Paraplegia. 1991;29:490–4.

© Springer International Publishing AG 2017
J.J. Wyndaele, A. Kovindha, *Urodynamic Testing After Spinal Cord Injury*,
DOI 10.1007/978-3-319-54900-2

Further Bibliography: Urodynamics and Related Topics

Stoehrer M, Goepel M, Kondo A, Kramer G, Madersbacher H, Millard R, et al. The standardization of terminology in neurogenic lower urinary tract dysfunction with some suggestions for diagnostic procedures. Neurourol Urodyn. 1999;18:139–58.

Abrams P, Cardozo L, Fall M, Griffiths D, Rosier P, Ulmsten U, et al. The standardisation of terminology of lower urinary tract function: report from the standardisation sub-committee of the International Continence Society. Neurourol Urodyn. 2002;21:167–78.

Schäfer W, Abrams P, Liao L, Mattiasson A, Pesce P, Spangberg A, et al. Good urodynamic practices: uroflowmetry, filling cystometry, and pressure-flow studies. Neurourol Urodyn. 2002;21:261–74.

Blaivas JG, Sinha HP, Zayed AA, Labib KB. Detrusor-sphincter dyssynergia: a detailed EMG study. J Urol. 1981;125:535–48.

Pannek J, Nehiba M. Morbidity of urodynamic testing to patients with spinal cord injury: is antibiotic prophylaxis necessary? Spinal Cord. 2007;45:771–4.

International Spinal Cord Data Sets

Biering-Sørensen F, Craggs M, Kennelly M, Schick E, Wyndaele JJ. International urodynamic basic spinal cord injury data set. Spinal Cord. 2008;46:513–6.

Biering-Sørensen F, Craggs M, Kennelly M, Schick E, Wyndaele JJ. International urinary tract imaging basic spinal cord injury data set. Spinal Cord. 2009;47:379–83.

Goetz LL, Cardenas DD, Kennelly M, Bonne Lee BS, Linsenmeyer T, Moser C, et al. International spinal cord injury urinary tract infection basic data set. Spinal Cord. 2013;51:700–4.

Neurogenic Bladder

Madersbacher H, Wyndaele JJ, Chartier-Kastler E, Fall M, Kovindha A, Perkash I, et al. Conservative management in the neuropathic patient. In: Abrams PKS, Wein A, editors. Incontinence. Paris: Health Publication Ltd; 1999. p. 775–812.

Madersbacher H, Wyndaele JJ, Igawa Y, Chancellor M, Chartier-Kastler E, Kovindha A. Conservative management in neuropathic urinary incontinence. In: Abrams P, Cardozo L, Khoury S, Wein A, editors. Incontinence. 2nd ed. Plymouth: Health Publication Ltd; 2002. p. 697–754.

Wyndaele JJ, Kovindha A, Madersbacher H, Radziszewski P, Ruffion A, Schurch B. Neurologic urinary and faecal incontinence. In: Abrams P, Cardozo L, Khoury S, Wein A, editors. Incontinence. 4th ed. Paris: Health Publication Ltd; 2009. p. 793–960.

Everaert K, Lumen N, Kerckhaert W, Willaert P, van Driel M. Urinary tract infections in spinal cord injury: prevention and treatment guidelines. Acta Clin Belg. 2009;64(4):335–40.

Biering-Sørensen F, Charlifue S, DeVivo M, Noonan V, Post M, Stripling T, et al. International spinal cord injury data sets. Spinal Cord. 2006;44(9):530–4.

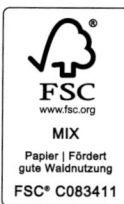

Zeitfracht Medien GmbH
Ferdinand-Jühlke-Straße 7
99095 Erfurt, Deutschland
produktsicherheit@kolibri360.de